# What Makes a Good Healthcare System?

# Comparisons, values, drivers

## Alan Gillies

*Professor of Information Management*
*Lancashire Postgraduate School of Medicine and Health*

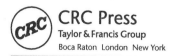

## CRC Press
Taylor & Francis Group
Boca Raton  London  New York

CRC Press is an imprint of the
Taylor & Francis Group, an **informa** business

First published 2003 by Radcliffe Publishing

Published 2016 by CRC Press
Taylor & Francis Group
6000 Broken Sound Parkway NW, Suite 300
Boca Raton, FL 33487-2742

© 2003 Alan Gillies
CRC Press is an imprint of Taylor & Francis Group, an Informa business

No claim to original U.S. Government works

ISBN-13: 978-1-85775-921-1 (pbk)

**Visit the Taylor & Francis Web site at
http://www.taylorandfrancis.com**

**and the CRC Press Web site at
http://www.crcpress.com**

British Library Cataloguing in Publication Data

A catalogue record for this book is available from the British Library.

Typeset by Advance Typesetting Ltd, Oxfordshire

# Contents

# Preface

Please read this bit!

This book is designed to meet two conflicting goals:

- to be readable and interesting enough to be read by anyone interested in health and healthcare
- to be rigorous and evidence based sufficient to be taken seriously by my academic peers.

There's actually no reason why a rigorous and well-argued book has to be boring and impenetrable. The problem is how to present the supporting evidence in such a way that it doesn't get in the way of the argument being presented. The solution that I have adopted is to publish a website with the book that provides links to as much evidence as possible in support of the main text. The website is found at http://www.goodhealthcare.org.uk.

If you just want to read the book, then ignore the references and further information and simply read it as a narrative. Alternatively, if you want to review the evidence then you will need an Internet browser.

Alan Gillies
*May 2003*

# Acknowledgements

I would like to thank many people for their help in this work:

- the Leverhulme Trust for the grant which enabled me to carry out the research
- the University of Central Lancashire and especially Professor Peter Aggett for supporting me in the operation of the research
- the RMIT Centre for Quality Management Research and especially Professor John Dalrymple and Warren Staples for hosting me during the Australian legs of the research
- Radcliffe Medical Press and especially Gill Nineham for commissioning and publishing the book
- all those people who gave freely of their time to talk to me and generously pointed me to sources of material, who are simply too numerous to mention but to whom I am incredibly grateful
- Professor Jan Davies for her detailed comments on the draft manuscript, particularly in the light of the fact that I know she doesn't agree with all my assertions and conclusions.

Finally, in spite of the above, I take full responsibility for the final text for whom no one else can be blamed!

# Acronyms and abbreviations

| Abbreviation | Meaning |
|---|---|
| A&E | Accident and emergency |
| ACT | Australian Capital Territory |
| AHCAs | Australian Health Care Arrangements |
| AIHW | Australian Institute of Health and Welfare, Government agency responsible for collating waiting time data |
| AMA | Australian Medical Association |
| AMI | Acute myocardial infarction |
| ARIA | Australian Remoteness Index |
| ASW | Approved social workers |
| BMA | British Medical Association |
| BMJ | British Medical Journal |
| BMMS | Better Medication Management System. Australian national prescribing record system |
| CCAC | Community Care Access Centre |
| CEO | Chief Executive Officer |
| CHD | Coronary heart disease |
| CHERA | Canadian Health Economics Research Association |
| CHI | Commission for Health Improvement |
| CHST | Canada Health and Social Transfer |
| CIHI | Canadian Institute of Health Information |
| CME | Continuing medical education |
| CPA | Care programme approach |
| CPD | Continuing professional development |
| CPN | Community psychiatric nurses |
| CQI | Continuous quality improvement |
| DoH | Department of Health. Responsible for healthcare in England and Wales |
| ECT | Electro convulsive therapy |
| EDT | Emergency duty team |
| EHCSP | Extended Health Care Services Program (Canada) |
| EHR | Electronic health record |
| EPF | Established programs financing (Canada) |
| FED | Front End Deductible (Australian health insurance product) |
| FP | For profit |
| GDP | Gross domestic product |
| GMC | General Medical Council (UK) |
| GP | General practitioner. This is used in the UK and Australian sense of a family doctor or family physician |
| HECS | Higher Education Contribution Scheme |
| HIC | Health Insurance Commission (Australia) |
| HoNOS | *Health of the Nation* outcome scores |

| | |
|---|---|
| HSC | Health Sciences Centre, Winnipeg |
| HSO | Health Service Organization (Canada) |
| HTF | Health Transition Fund (Canada) |
| ICU | Intensive care unit |
| IHST | Intensive Home Support Team |
| IT | Information technology |
| MMR | Vaccine for mumps, measles and rubella |
| NAW | National Assembly for Wales |
| NFP | Not for profit |
| NHS | National Health Service |
| NICE | National Institute for Clinical Excellence |
| NICU | Neonatal intensive care unit |
| NPSA | National Patient Safety Agency |
| NSF | National Service Framework |
| NSW | New South Wales (Australian state) |
| NT | Northern Territory (Australian state) |
| OECD | Office for Economic Cooperation and Development |
| OFHN | Ontario family health network |
| OMA | Ontario Medical Association |
| OT | Occupational therapist |
| PBS | Pharmaceutical Benefits Scheme, Australian national Pharma-care programme |
| PCG | Primary care group |
| PCN | Primary care network (Canada) |
| PCT | Primary care trust |
| PFI | Private Finance Initiative |
| PHC | Primary healthcare |
| PIP | Practice Incentives Program |
| PRODIGY | A prescribing decision support system |
| PROFESS | A monitoring system to be used with PRODIGY |
| Qld | Queensland (Australian state) |
| RACGP | Royal Australian College of General Practitioners |
| SA | South Australia (Australian state) |
| SID | social information database |
| StBOP | Shifting the Balance of Power in the NHS |
| Tas. | Tasmania (Australian state) |
| TEACH | Telecentres for Education and Community Health (Canada) |
| UK | United Kingdom. Non-UK readers, please note that the NHS in Scotland and Northern Ireland is organised differently from England and Wales |
| VCHC | Variety Children's Heart Centre. Cardiac surgery centre in Winnipeg |
| Vic. | Victoria (Australian state) |
| WA | Western Australia (Australian state) |
| WHO | World Health Organization |

---

# CHAPTER I

# People in their daily lives

## About this book

Health is a very political issue in today's world. Politicians talk a lot about improving the healthcare system in their countries. They assume that they know what is a better system. They may even assume that they know how to make their system better. This book sets out to challenge these assumptions. It seeks to examine our assumptions about what is a 'good' system. It will do this by comparing three national systems from the United Kingdom (UK), Australia and Canada.

In each country, there is a different view of what a good healthcare system is trying to achieve. We shall consider these from the perspective of the current situation in each country, the policy documents which tell us where each country is trying to get to, and comments gathered from key stakeholders to introduce a note of reality.

However, before we get to our analysis of each country, we must establish a basis for our comparison. To start this we shall consider the needs of patients through four different individuals with diverse needs and expectations.

## Andrew, 35, stressed-out executive

Andrew lives in Guildford, but works in London. He works typically 50 to 60 hours a week. This leaves him fairly tired and stressed, with little time for exercise. He considers himself to be careful about his health. Accordingly, he has reduced his smoking to 15 cigarettes a day, and restricts himself to one glass of whisky in an evening on his return home. He shares a bottle of wine with Jane, his wife, most Friday and some Saturday nights. He avoids food he considers unhealthy, such as fish and chips, hamburgers and the like. On mid-week evenings, he often eats pre-packaged meals if Jane is out.

Every so often, he fits in a game of squash with his best friend Gareth and walks to the station occasionally in the summer when he has time.

He has not had a day off from the office for ill health in the past ten years, and has not visited his general practitioner (GP) in that time. He did receive a letter from his GP inviting him to attend for a consultation last year, but did not consider it important enough to make space in his diary.

## Anna, 15, teenager

Anna lives in Doncaster and is a healthy, active teenager who likes going out with her mates at the weekend. She worries about her weight and whether she is overweight.

She is a vegetarian and eats a lot of salads. If she is feeling anxious about her weight, she will skip lunch.

She has been seeing the same boy for two months, and although she is not sexually active, thinks that her boyfriend Mike would like them to be.

She has only visited her doctor with her Mum, and does not know the name of her registered GP. She thinks that doctors are for when you are ill. There is a female GP in her practice, but she doesn't know if she's allowed to go and speak to her, and if so, whether you can do this if you're not ill.

## Harold, 75, old-age pensioner

Harold lives in Birmingham. He lives alone since his wife died a few years ago. He has difficulty getting about because of an arthritic hip. He is on the list for a replacement, but he has been waiting for nine months and he doesn't yet know when he will get his operation. Meals on Wheels call three times a week to provide a hot meal and check on him. He gave up smoking ten years ago when he had problems with angina. He has a sweet tooth and likes cakes and biscuits. His old doctor retired six years ago and he was transferred to a newly qualified female doctor who he finds it more difficult to talk to. His children have moved away and the rest of his family are back in Jamaica, which Harold left back in the early 1960s when he came to England to look for work.

## Daphne, 32, schoolteacher

Daphne lives in Northampton. She recently married David. They have been living together for eight years and have decided to start a family. Daphne has been preparing for pregnancy by stopping smoking and confining her drinking to a couple of glasses of dry white wine on a Friday night. She went to her doctor's surgery for advice about the planned pregnancy, and instead of speaksing to her usual (male) doctor, she talked to one of the female partners in the practice.

## Health needs

Each of our four characters has diverse needs.

Andrew considers himself to be basically healthy and health conscious. He sees the fact that he has not been to the GP for ten years as a measure of his health. He has taken steps to eliminate those factors placing him most at risk; he has cut down on his smoking, drinks moderately by his judgement and avoids high-fat foods. He looks on his exercise as positive, but thinks he does more than he actually does.

In reality, his smoking is still a risk factor and his drinking is probably too high. Home measures are notoriously large, so his nightly whisky is probably two to three units of alcohol per day and his weekly wine intake may add up to 12 units. This puts him between 26 and 33 units a week, which is at a level where problems may occur.

His exercise is too sporadic to be useful, and sudden bursts of exercise such as squash may be actually harmful. His diet, whilst not bad, seems unlikely to provide sufficient fruit and vegetables and may well be high in salt due to the pre-packaged meals, which may also provide too much fat.

Whilst none of these factors make it likely that he will drop dead tomorrow, they would be risk factors if combined with other factors such as:

- raised blood pressure
- family history of heart disease
- family history of diabetes.

In reality, Andrew is a fairly typical male in their thirties. The fact that he has neither the inclination nor the time to visit his GP to establish any level of risk means that he could be ignorant of the real level of risk.

Anna is much more health conscious in her own way. She receives much advice from reading teenage magazines and believes that her diet is helping her keep her weight down, which is a priority for her. Whilst she does not have an eating disorder, anxieties over putting on weight are likely to take priority over eating a balanced diet. As a vegetarian she may be deficient in protein and also some key nutrients. Living at home, where her mum makes limited provision for her vegetarianism, may exacerbate this problem.

Anna also recognises a need for access and advice on contraception and possibly in broader matters to do with her relationship. In the absence of understanding or feeling able to access the formal healthcare system, she is likely to use more informal modes of advice – peers, magazines etc. – and possibly less than ideal or no contraception if she decides to sleep with her boyfriend.

Harold has more traditional healthcare needs. He needs an operation, and is currently waiting for the procedure. His limited mobility, in the mean time, creates other care needs and reduces his quality of life. It will force him into a sedentary life-style, which may create other health problems. His sweet tooth may put him at risk of diabetes, and the risks arising from a diabetic coma for an elderly man living alone are significant.

His colour and ethnic background, together with his inability to relate to his new GP, may also create barriers and prevent him accessing all the healthcare advice and services that he might need.

Daphne has adopted a planned approach to her pregnancy. She has taken advice from both her GP practice and other more informal sources such as books, magazines and her friends. She has an increased awareness of health issues because of the impact upon her baby. She is also aware that the proposed pregnancy will have a major impact on her own body. In contrast to Andrew, who is of similar age, she has been in regular contact with the healthcare system due to her use of the contraceptive pill in the past and her cervical smears, which she has been having done regularly. As part of the checks for her repeat prescription of the contraceptive pill, she has received checks on her blood pressure.

For now, we will leave Andrew, Anna, Harold and Daphne in their respective lives, but we shall return to them later.

# Quality as a measure of 'goodness'

When we talk of defining how good a healthcare system is, we generally do this in terms of quality assurance. Quality assurance is the process of measuring performance against a defined standard and seeing how it compares. This idea has its origins in engineering and science where defining standards can be relatively straightforward.

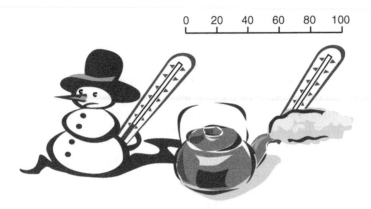

**Figure 1.1**

Consider the measurement of temperature. In order to measure temperature, first we plunge our thermometer in melting ice. We can mark the mercury level as 0°C. Similarly, we can place it in a cloud of steam and mark this as 100°C. We then divide the difference by 100 to make our temperature scale. This forms the basis of an internationally agreed scale of 'hotness' which is consistent and objective.

In science and engineering, it is sometimes possible to measure quality in this objective way. For example, the quality of a batch of ball-bearings may reasonably be defined in terms of a simple set of physical parameters:

- diameter
- roundness
- metallurgical composition
- hardness.

For each of these parameters, we can agree acceptable ranges and measure whether each individual ball-bearing meets the requirements.

There are times when it is suggested that we can measure the quality of healthcare in the same way. We can't. But there is a more fundamental problem. The scientists have a consensus over what temperature is. It is a measure of 'hotness'. In quantitative terms, it is a measure of the kinetic energy of the molecules making up whatever you are measuring the temperature of.

If we move to our ball-bearing example, things are a little less clear. Standards may now be defined in terms of a range of parameters. The relative importance of each parameter may vary according to context, but each can be measured objectively, and frankly the relative importance is not likely to be controversial.

In healthcare the measures are often not objective, and the relative importance is both critical and may well be controversial.

To take one example, consider Harold and his hip operation. How shall we measure the quality of this procedure? Here is a range of measures that are used in practice:

- How long does Harold have to wait to see a specialist who decides he needs an operation?
- How long does Harold have to wait once the specialist decides he needs an operation?
- How many people like Harold are treated in his local hospital each year?
- How many people like Harold have to wait to be treated more than one year?
- How likely is Harold to catch an infection whilst in hospital for his operation?
- How likely is Harold to be readmitted as a result of catching an infection whilst in hospital for his operation?
- How many days will Harold have to spend in hospital to have his operation?

Here is a range of measures that may not be used, but might be of more use to Harold:

- How much mobility will Harold get back after the operation?
- How long will it take him to recover from the operation itself?
- How long will it take him to get used to his new hip?
- How often will someone visit to check if he's OK whilst he's recovering?

Now multiply this by all the Harolds, Daphnes, Annas and Andrews in the country, all their health needs, add the resource constraints of any healthcare system and you start to appreciate the complexity of measuring the quality of healthcare.

The purpose of this book is to ask the question: 'What is a good healthcare system?' If we are able to answer this question in a sensible way, then we can start to measure performance against our model of a good system.

# The idea of a gold standard

In traditional quality assurance, we measure things against an accepted standard. For example, traditionally, mass in kilograms was measured against a lump of metal weighing 1 kg (nowadays, the standard is stated in terms of the mass containing a huge number of atoms).

The phrase 'gold standard' was originally defined as the use of gold as the standard value for the money of a country. If a country will redeem any of its money in gold it is said to be using the gold standard. The United States of America (USA) and many other Western countries adhered to the gold standard during the early 1900s. However, the UK abandoned the gold standard in 1931 and the USA abandoned it in 1971. The colloquial use of the term remains and it is used to express the idea of the highest possible quality, against which all quality may be measured.

For health, there is simply no gold standard. This is due to a number of reasons, including:

- *Any healthcare system is doomed to ultimate failure.* We all die in the end and cannot stay healthy forever, nor can we always expect to recover from illness. Any sense of a reference standard can only be relative.
- *Since reference standards in healthcare are relative, they depend upon expectation.* Patients have expectations of care and will define the quality of their experience accordingly. For example, suppose you want to see your family doctor today. You might have any of the following expectations:
  - you may expect to see your choice of doctor today
  - you may expect to be able to see a doctor today, but be prepared to wait to see the doctor of your choice
  - you may be happy to see a practice nurse today, but be prepared to wait to see the doctor of your choice
  - you may believe that your family doctor is a busy man and be prepared to wait till tomorrow to see him with no alternative offered.

  In the UK and Canada, we expect to be able to do this for free. In Australia, there may be an expectation that in order to see the doctor of your choice, you will have to pay. The quality of the service provided as perceived by the patient is whether their expectation is met, rather than whether some absolute standard is met.

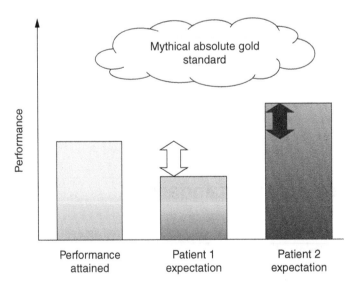

**Figure 1.2** Patient expectations.

In the simple case shown in Figure 1.2, patient 1's expectations have been exceeded but patient 2, who received the same standard of care, is disappointed because their expectations have not been met.

- *There are different stakeholders in the situation.* The clinician may have a view on how many patients they can see in a day; their colleagues may also have a view on whether they are pulling their weight within a partnership situation; the funding body in a public system may have a view as to whether the service provides good value for money.

In order to start to appraise these issues and others, we shall consider two case studies in the next chapter based around Daphne and Harold.

# CHAPTER 2

# People meet the healthcare system: two case studies

## Daphne has a baby

Twelve months on, and Daphne is about to have a baby. She feels as if she's in a play and there is a large number of characters:

The Cast

| | |
|---|---|
| Daphne | The mother |
| Baby | Not yet born, referred to throughout by the healthcare professionals as 'Baby' |
| David | Baby's father and Daphne's husband |
| Susan | A hospital midwife |
| Mr Khan | The hospital consultant |
| Dr Jones | A female GP from Daphne's practice |
| Dr Taylor | Daphne's registered GP |
| Sarah Carr | The midwifery unit manager |

## Daphne (the mother)

Daphne's view of the quality of her experience will depend upon two factors: a successful outcome and a positive experience before, during and after the birth. The duality of this view is emphasised by the fact that most mothers are not ill.

Obviously at some points, these views are reinforcing. A simple and successful birth will encourage a positive view of the whole experience. However, some procedures, which may be deemed clinically desirable to maximise the probability of a successful outcome, may be highly invasive and disturbing for the mother.

During the birth, Daphne is asked to give consent to a probe being put into Baby's scalp to monitor Baby's heartbeat. She agrees to the procedure but wishes someone would explain why it is necessary and worries that something might be wrong, as well as finding the whole procedure painful.

## Baby

Baby, although unable to express a view, is the focus of at least half the care provided. We know little of Baby's actual experience of birth, and are unable to gain informed consent! Obviously it is traumatic, and additional invasive procedures will add to the trauma. Equally, Baby wants to make it into the world fit and healthy.

## David (Baby's father and Daphne's husband)

David has a dual role as father and husband. He is unsure of his roles and feels that although he wants to share in the whole experience, he will be excluded if a crisis should happen. When consulted about putting the probe into Baby's scalp, he feels that it is probably unnecessary and done to protect the hospital, rather than Daphne or Baby. However, he feels that to vocalise these thoughts would be to appear cavalier about the health of his wife and baby, and therefore does not object.

## Susan (the hospital midwife)

Susan, the hospital midwife, is responsible for the delivery of the baby. She sees her prime responsibility as a successful outcome for mother and baby. Her view of quality is complicated by her dual responsibility to both mother and baby. She feels that her care for patients is being increasingly influenced by a need to demonstrate that all eventualities were considered in the light of possible litigation in the event of problems. She knows of three colleagues who have had complaints made against them in spite of the fact that they believed they acted in good faith.

## Mr Khan (the hospital consultant)

Mr Khan has seen Daphne twice during her pregnancy. He will become directly involved in the birth only if there are clinical complications. One of his female colleagues once remarked that this made her an awful expectant mother as she had only ever witnessed difficult births. This, coupled with the fact that he carries ultimate responsibility for any clinical problems, means that Mr Khan sees Daphne's pregnancy primarily as a clinical episode. When challenged by one of the midwives recently, he replied that it was his job to prepare for the worst and hope for the best, by anticipating all the problems that might occur and thereby reducing the risks of them actually occurring and having serious implications for Daphne and her baby.

## Dr Jones (a female GP from Daphne's practice)

Dr Caroline Jones has seen Daphne before and during the pregnancy. She will visit Daphne after the birth. She has no direct involvement in the birth itself.

## Dr Taylor (Daphne's registered GP)

Dr John Taylor is the GP with whom Daphne is registered. It is likely that he will become Baby's registered GP as well. He has been briefed on Daphne's pregnancy by Caroline but has had no direct involvement in Daphne's care.

## Sarah Carr (the midwifery unit manager)

Sarah Carr is the manager of the unit and has the job of ensuring the quality of patient care delivered. Crucially, she has to weigh the needs of all patients rather than individuals. She also has to weigh decisions against available resources and this leads to having to evaluate the quality of care against the quantity. She is under pressure to meet targets set by the hospital and the Government, which do not always seem to be realistic or the most relevant to individual mothers like Daphne.

## What happened next?

Against the apparent trend towards elective Caesareans, Daphne had a healthy baby boy by vaginal delivery.

## Discussion from this case study

Childbirth is not an illness and there has been a vocal campaign to keep the process as natural as possible. In spite of this, the number of elective Caesareans is still rising in the UK (*see* Figure 2.1) and appears to have caught up with other countries (*see* Table 2.1).[1]

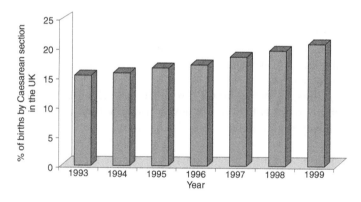

**Figure 2.1**   Caesarean rates in the UK since 1993.[1]

**Table 2.1**   Percentage of births delivered by Caesarean section[1]

| | *Percentage of births delivered by Caesarean section (1999)*[1] |
|---|---|
| USA | 22.0% |
| UK | 20.4% |
| Canada | 18.9% |
| Australia | 21.1% |

As recently as 1996, the percentage of births by Caesarean section in the UK lagged behind those in Canada, but have since overtaken (*see* Figure 2.2).[1]

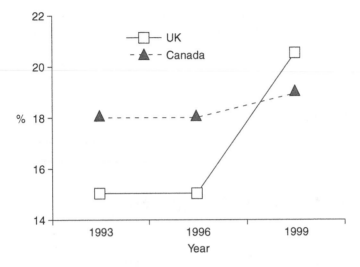

**Figure 2.2** Caesarean rates in the UK have overtaken Canada since 1996.[1]

Daphne's experience was different from those of mothers in other countries. When I was talking to an expectant father from Alberta in Canada, he was appalled at the lack of routine medical intervention in the process in the UK. He regarded it as absolutely essential that the whole procedure was supervised directly by an obstetrician.

Australian interviewees, including GPs, regarded the UK general practice system as too restrictive on patient choice, believing that the kind of choice exercised by Daphne was simply not available in the UK system:

> I think it's disgraceful that UK patients can't choose their GP.
>
> Australian GP

Conversely, Australian midwives have been reduced to a minor role in the birth itself by the difficulty in obtaining indemnity insurance. This would be regarded as a major loss of choice by UK mothers-to-be.

The clinical outcomes in the three countries are broadly similar. The UK has shown dramatic improvements in infant and maternal mortality rates in the past 30 years. However, it still lags behind Australia and Canada in the last available data (*see* Table 2.2).

The problem for any policy maker is how to balance the needs of mothers such as Daphne who need minimal medical intervention, with the need to protect mothers and babies whose health may be at genuine and high risk.

**Table 2.2** Maternal mortality rates for major countries (Source: Hill *et al.*)[2]

| Country | Adjusted maternal mortality rates |
|---------|-----------------------------------|
| Australia | 6 |
| Canada | 6 |
| UK | 10 |
| Germany | 12 |
| Japan | 12 |
| US | 12 |
| France | 20 |

# Harold gets his hip operation

Meanwhile, Harold has reached the top of the waiting list for his operation. He has a similar list of actors in his story:

| | |
|---|---|
| Harold | The patient |
| Mr Wilson | Orthopaedic surgeon at Harold's local hospital |
| Dr Taylor | Anaesthetist at Harold's local hospital |
| Irene | Harold's designated social worker |
| David Watson | The general surgery manager |

## Harold (the patient)

Harold is pleased that he has finally reached the top of the list for his operation. On the other hand he is anxious about going into hospital. He is concerned both about the strangeness of the environment and the fact that several of his friends went into hospital and did not come out again.

## Mr Wilson (orthopaedic surgeon at Harold's local hospital)

Mr Wilson has been carrying out additional operations to get the waiting list down. However, he is finding the extra work tiring, particularly as he seeks to keep up his private work. He visits Harold the evening before the operation to reassure him about the procedure and answer his questions.

## Dr Taylor (anaesthetist at Harold's local hospital)

In view of Harold's age and general state of health, including his history of angina, Dr Taylor is taking particular care over the anaesthesia for Harold's operation. He has met with Mr Wilson to discuss the particular issues before surgery starts.

## Irene (Harold's designated social worker)

Irene is pleased that Harold is able to have the operation. Her concern is with his post-operative care. The local press has been running stories about patients being discharged quickly from hospital with consequent complications and potential readmission. Irene regards Harold as particularly at risk due to the absence of any supportive family network.

## David Watson (the general surgery manager)

The priority for David has been to reduce his waiting lists and waiting times. The hospital has looked at use of operating theatres, discharge times and bed occupancy rates. Although there has been an increase in readmission rates following earlier release of patients in an attempt to increase throughput, this is lower on David's list of priorities than the headline waiting time indicators.

# Discussion from this case study

There is no doubt that one of the biggest weaknesses of the UK National Health Service (NHS) has been access to secondary care, and procedures such as hip operations have been some of the worst affected.

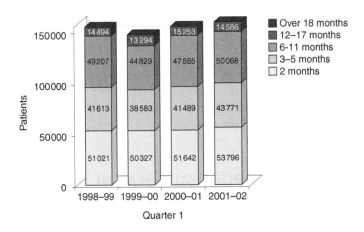

**Figure 2.3** Number of patients on orthopaedic waiting lists in England.[3]

Figure 2.3 shows that in spite of the Government's best efforts, in England in 2001 there were over 50 000 patients awaiting orthopaedic operations who, like Harold, had been waiting more than six months, over 14 500 who had been waiting more than 12 months, and for the first time since 1998 there were patients who had been waiting more than 18 months (46 of them!).

However, in fairness to the UK NHS, it does at least have a systematic monitoring system and a view of the scale of the problem. Contrast this with Canada, where one person commented that 'waiting lists on the scale of the UK would bring down a Provincial Government' and others expressed similar views. But there does not appear to be any way to reliably measure the extent of the problem:[4]

> With rare exceptions, waiting lists in Canada, as in most countries, are non-standardized, capriciously organized, poorly monitored and (according to most informed observers) in grave need of retooling. As such most of those currently in use are at best misleading sources of data on access to care, and at worst instruments of misinformation, propaganda and general mischief.

For the first time, in 2001 Statistics Canada produced an overall figure for waiting times available by province. The figure is defined as the distribution of waiting times for non-emergency surgeries, based upon the household population aged 15 and over (*see* Table 2.3).

**Table 2.3**  Waiting time in Canada in 2001[5]

| Waiting time for non-emergency surgeries | Number of persons | % |
|---|---|---|
| Less than 1 month | 457 133 | 39.5 |
| 1 to 3 months | 478 233 | 41.3 |
| Longer than 3 months | 221 674 | 19.2 |

The waiting lists in Australia are reported by the Australian Institute of Health and Welfare (AIHW), a government agency. Whilst they are not reported in exactly the same way as in the UK, the percentage of patients waiting more than 12 months for orthopaedic surgery is shown in Table 2.4.

**Table 2.4**  Waiting times for orthopaedic surgery by state in 2001 (Source: AIHW)[6]

| State | Percentage of patients waiting more than 12 months for orthopaedic surgery |
|---|---|
| New South Wales | 10.3 |
| Victoria | 7.7 |
| Queensland | 3.5 |
| Western Australia | 13.9 |
| South Australia | 8.3 |
| Tasmania | 21.1 |
| Australian Capital Territory | 4.5 |
| Northern Territory | 6.6 |
| Total | 8.2 |

The comparable figure for England, derived from the Department of Health data,[3] is 9.0%. This is just worse than the Australian average, but better than a number of Australian provinces, including New South Wales. This is at odds with the perception of those Australians whom I talked to, who expressed the view that their system provided significantly better access to care than the UK NHS.

However, further investigation shows that whilst most waiting times in the UK are broadly similar across specialities, in Australia many are doing much better than in orthopaedics, so in most areas Harold could expect to be seen much more quickly (*see* Figure 2.4).

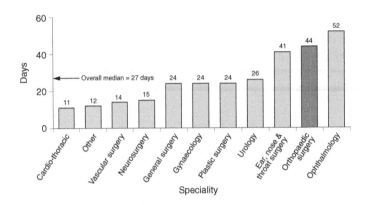

**Figure 2.4** Median waiting times by speciality.[7]

Interestingly, comparing the overall situation in Canada and Australia shows that Australia treats 50% of its patients within 27 days, whereas Canada manages 40% within one month. However, it should be remembered that:

- differences between provinces/states and speciality mean that this overall difference is much less than the variation within each national system
- definitions of waiting times are notoriously variable, in terms of when the clock starts ticking.

Recent efforts in the UK have led to a reduction in some waiting times. However, this has led to concerns over the quality of care offered, especially in the case of vulnerable patients such as Harold. Lengths of stay in hospital have reduced dramatically and whilst this has been due partly to improved surgical techniques reducing post-operative trauma, there are also concerns over the pressure to release beds for the next patient.

In the next chapter, we start to consider these and other issues on a system-wide basis. However, the ultimate merit of any system remains the impact of the system upon the lives of individuals in promoting health and dealing with illness as it occurs.

# CHAPTER 3

# What is a good healthcare system?

## Introduction

Any healthcare system may be defined as a collection of encounters between people. At its simplest, the encounter is between a patient or care recipient and a professional or care-giver. However, as we have seen, each stakeholder in those encounters has their own perspective, and the reality is that each encounter is part of a series of encounters with a complex range of stakeholders.

In spite of the fact that many of the key characteristics of a healthy population and a successful care system are determined by what goes on in those individual encounters, decisions about planning and policy are necessarily made at the macroscopic level. In particular, decisions taken at the macroscopic level tend to be about prioritisation within the healthcare system. Few politicians are prepared to speak of the rationing of healthcare, but in reality all systems have finite resources, so planning decisions are as much about deciding what is not going to happen as what is. The challenges facing any healthcare system may therefore be represented in terms of a series of conflicts pulling the system in different directions.

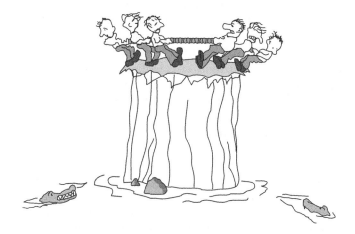

Figure 3.1   A series of conflicts pulling the system in different directions.

# Health or illness?

It was George Orwell in his famous novel *1984*[8] who pointed out that traditionally Government departments have names opposed to their real purpose. In most countries, the traditional focus of the Department of Health has been to manage illness rather than to achieve health.

Progress towards a more enlightened view may be traced to the widespread adoption of the 1978 Alma-Ata Declaration,[9] which emphasised primary healthcare:

> Primary healthcare is essential healthcare based on practical, scientific-ally sound and socially acceptable methods and technology made universally accessible to individuals and families in the community through their full participation and at a cost that the community and country can afford to maintain at every stage of their development in the spirit of self-reliance and self-determination. It forms an integral part both of the country's health system, of which it is the central function and main focus, and of the overall social and economic development of the community. It is the first level of contact of individuals, the family and community with the national health system bringing healthcare as close as possible to where people live and work, and constitutes the first element of a continuing healthcare process.
>
> **VII**
> Primary healthcare:
>
> 1 reflects and evolves from the economic conditions and sociocultural and political characteristics of the country and its communities and is based on the application of the relevant results of social, biomedical and health services research and public health experience;
> 2 addresses the main health problems in the community, providing pro-motive, preventive, curative and rehabilitative services accordingly;
> 3 includes at least: education concerning prevailing health problems and the methods of preventing and controlling them; promotion of food supply and proper nutrition; an adequate supply of safe water and basic sanitation; maternal and child healthcare, including family planning; immunization against the major infectious diseases; pre-vention and control of locally endemic diseases; appropriate treatment of common diseases and injuries; and provision of essential drugs.
>
> All governments should formulate national policies, strategies and plans of action to launch and sustain primary healthcare as part of a comprehensive national health system and in coordination with other sectors. To this end, it will be necessary to exercise political will, to mobilize the country's resources and to use available external resources rationally.

On the twentieth anniversary, the World Health Organization (WHO) was able to claim major advances in health:

> Since the PHC approach was enshrined, the worldwide infant mortality rate has decreased from 90 per 1000 live births in 1975 to 59 in 1995 – a decrease of 34% – while immunization coverage for children under one year of age has risen from 20% to 80% between 1980 and 1990. In the mid 1970s, only 38% of the people in developing countries had access to safe drinking water and 32% to adequate sanitation, whereas those figures had risen to 66% and 53%, respectively, by 1990.

As will be seen later, this health improvement is not restricted to developing countries. In spite of this, many national systems seem to be focused on hospitals, which are, as one wag put it, 'places where people who are wound down go to wind up'.[10] The UK has one of the strongest emphases upon primary healthcare and its health promotion role. The reasons for this are discussed in Chapter 6 on the UK NHS.

Prevention of disease and promotion of health is in theory a win–win situation. It is cheaper to prevent disease than treat it; it is also better for the person to remain healthy than get sick and then recover. However, in the real world, two factors sour this idyllic picture.

- *Disjointed budgeting.* In most healthcare systems, the budgets for health promotion and primary care are kept separate. Thus increased costs in primary care are often offset by savings in secondary care, but these are not seen together. An example cited by a UK interviewee was the case of steroid inhalers for asthma sufferers. Greatly increased prescribing of such medications has contributed to a rise in drug costs. There is good evidence that this cost is much less than the cost of emergency admissions arising from a failure to prescribe. Thus what is a benefit in health and financial terms is not seen as such and general practitioners may be criticised for their apparently profligate behaviour. This situation may be distorted further if different parts of the system are on opposite sides of a public/private divide. Thus in Canada, the situation is distorted in the other direction by the fact that the hospital costs are met from public funding, whereas drug costs are met from private funds.
- *Voter recognition.* As stated earlier, health is a highly emotive political issue. Voters do not recognise that their healthcare system is doing a good job if it helps them stay healthy: they do not notice the system at all. The quality and availability of care when people are ill is a much more visible indicator of quality to voters. Politicians who make decisions about healthcare priorities may be influenced by their need to achieve re-election in a relatively short time.

Historically, all the great advances in health have been caused by prevention of diseases, including as highlights:

- provision of clean water
- eradication of polio and cholera
- reductions in smoking in developed countries at least.

# Health or healthcare?

Given the above, there is another question, which is 'How far can healthcare improve health?'

Health is a complex issue and many of the factors influencing overall health are either not in the traditional domain of healthcare or are difficult to influence, e.g.:

- water quality
- diet
- genetics
- consumption of alcohol, tobacco and narcotic drugs.

In reality, the two biggest reductions in killer diseases in the UK in the 1990s were as a direct result of healthcare interventions:

- reduction in cervical cancer deaths in women, due largely to systematic screening
- reduction in lung cancer deaths in men, due largely to reductions in smoking.

Neither screening nor anti-smoking campaigns can coerce people into a change in lifestyle, but the reality is that they are having a demonstrable impact on mortality rates. One significant problem with this sort of intervention is that it has an inequitable effect with poorer, more disadvantaged populations accessing services less frequently, and hence achieving less benefit. In countries with sparse rural populations such as Canada and Australia, the rural populations can be particularly disadvantaged since physicians are often reluctant to locate to these areas.

Interestingly, the NHS Direct telephone service in the UK appears to be quite successful in reaching socially disadvantaged populations:[11]

> People in social groups D and E are less likely to be aware of NHS Direct – 49 per cent against 61 per cent for the population as a whole. However, they are also more likely than average to see NHS Direct as a useful service (75 per cent against an average of 70 per cent).
>
> Indeed, preliminary research carried out in South East London indicates higher levels of usage of NHS Direct in council wards with high levels of social deprivation. This suggests that, if they can be made aware of the service and provided with access, this group are enthusiastic users of the service. Nine NHS Direct sites had no specific initiatives aimed at less advantaged social groups when we contacted them in June 2001.

However, sometimes the intervention of the system can have a negative effect. In the current furore over the measles–mumps–rubella (MMR) vaccine, the more the healthcare professionals seek to reassure parents that the vaccine is safe, the greater the opposition appears to be, and the greater the belief that there is some sort of cover-up going on. This may be an example of what Professor Bob Evans, the distinguished Canadian health economist, refers to as a 'zombie' idea:[12] an idea that will not die and the harder you knock it down, the sooner it appears to come back again to haunt you! Ultimately, it is impossible to prove a negative, and sometimes efforts to do so can be counter-productive. For example, at the height of the scare over the MMR, the *British Medical Journal* (*BMJ*) fast-tracked a paper[13] to publication. A group of healthcare professionals who were well disposed to the vaccine thought the evidence presented in this paper was poor and sent an electronic response to the *BMJ* to this effect (look at the electronic responses accompanying the article on the *BMJ* website). This apparently limited success in killing the zombie can resurrect it even more quickly!

# Health as quality of life

Traditionally, health has been viewed as the absence of disease, and healthcare as the treatment and increasingly the prevention of disease. This would seem to reflect a medical view of the world: health is being considered in a more holistic and positive sense.

One way of doing this is to consider health in terms of quality of life. Some of the most contentious issues arise from this view. In the UK, some of the longest waiting times for treatment arise from conditions that severely impair quality of life, e.g. cataracts and hip replacements.

In Canada, where waiting times are less, and crucially the Canada Health Act enshrines a patient's right to 'all medically necessary treatment free at the point of care', there are voices raised against this trend in a way that seems unlikely to be acceptable in the UK:[14]

> The medicalization of the human condition has reached an incredible level that is now almost certainly crossing the border between net benefits and net harm. Let's go through a few examples from birth to death, some of which would actually be laughable if they were not so serious. Medical care around childbirth has saved countless lives, but almost a third of women seem now to be either unable or unwilling to give birth without the surgeon's knife. We are in danger of destroying the wondrous benefits of antibiotics by giving them unnecessarily to so many children with minor respiratory infections ... baldness is now a disease for which people are urged to see their doctor.

On the other hand, many people will be more sympathetic to the complaints made about resuscitation where it is pointed out that resuscitation is the norm in the absence of written instructions to the contrary, even in cases of terminal disease.

The system can directly affect things here. In the Canadian system, where physicians are remunerated according to how much care you receive, there is an incentive to provide more services than is really necessary. In a capitation system such as the UK, there is an incentive to provide less treatment, or at least no incentive to provide more. In the UK, the private sector is often seen as providing either quicker access to treatment for conditions deemed to be having an adverse effect on quality of life, or surgery such as cosmetic surgery that may be deemed to be medically frivolous.

Canadians regard equity of access to 'medically essential services' as a cornerstone of their system. Whilst this is laudable, it does tend to focus the debate on what is medically essential and what is not.

# A model of a healthcare system

Faced with the variety of stakeholders and the different views of health and healthcare, we need to define a framework that can be used as a basis for discussion in the rest of this book.

Quality assurance is the usual model that is used to assess how good a healthcare system is. In this model, it is assumed that you can define what healthcare should be about and measure how good actual performance is relative to your target. For example, if you wish to eradicate a disease, there is a threshold level of immunisation beyond which the disease cannot propagate. Thus if vaccination rates exceed this threshold, then the entire population is protected. Targets such as this are clear and unambiguous.

In other areas, it is more difficult to measure the quality of care or to establish meaningful targets. Some goals will conflict with others. Consider the objective of equity. One of the objectives of the UK Government is to 'end the postcode lottery', or the inequity in access to care based upon where the patient lives.

At the same time, the biggest reform in the 1997 *New NHS* White Paper[15] was the establishment of locally based primary care groups (now evolved into primary care trusts) to meet the health needs of local populations. Therefore, local organisations will prioritise those conditions that have the greatest need in their area. If the Government forces these organisations to meet national standards across the board, then their ability to meet the specific needs of their populations will be severely restricted. Equity is traded against meeting local needs.

In this book, I shall take a step back from the traditional quality assurance mechanisms and look at the more fundamental question of 'what is the system trying to achieve?'

We may characterise what is being striven for as the underlying *values* of the system. These values may appear to be self-evident, but in practice they vary from country to country and culture to culture. However, whilst policy may start from underlying values, it is subject to being driven off course by external factors and constraints.

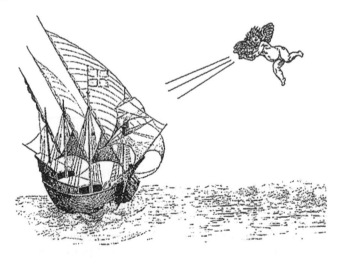

**Figure 3.2**   Policy may be established in terms of core values, but be driven off course by external factors and constraints.

Probably, the most common driver is finance, but policy is also driven by political ideology and in recent years has been driven by high-profile scandals in the UK and Canada. Therefore we represent policy as the result of values and drivers (*see* Figure 3.3).

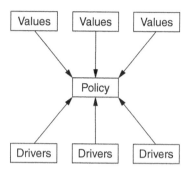

**Figure 3.3**   Policy is based upon values but driven by constraints.

In our model, we describe this in terms of the values of the national system. These are the aims of the system. Nowhere are such values more clearly stated than in the Canada Health Act:[16]

*Public administration*: requires that the administration and operation of the healthcare insurance plan of a province be carried out on a non-profit basis by a public authority responsible to the provincial government.

*Comprehensiveness*: requires that all medically necessary services provided by hospitals and doctors be covered under the provincial healthcare insurance plan.

*Universality*: requires that all residents of a province be entitled to public health-care insurance coverage.

*Accessibility*: requires reasonable access unimpeded by financial or other barriers to medically necessary hospital and physician services for residents, and reasonable compensation for both physicians and hospitals.

*Portability*: requires that coverage under public healthcare insurance be main-tained when a resident moves or travels within Canada or travels outside the country (coverage outside Canada is restricted to the coverage the resident has in his/her own province).

Defenders of the Canada Health Act defend these values with an evangelical zeal, and any attempt to debate these core values is met with blanket opposition, which may not be a bad thing. In practice, debate shifts to the application of these principles and to the precise definitions of terms such as 'medically necessary'. Furthermore, the provincial administration of healthcare provides a natural mechanism for diversity, with provinces such as Alberta making use of private facilities to deliver public healthcare in a manner which would be an anathema in other provinces.

Having established policy, it is necessary to implement that policy. The second half of our model deals with the implementation of the policy. Implementation is driven by goals and standards. Through these goals and standards, policy influences practice. The process of quality assurance is used to measure whether practice reflects the goals and standards set as a result of policy (*see* Figure 3.4).

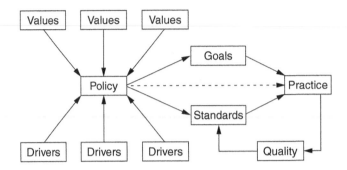

**Figure 3.4** The complete model.

In the next chapter, I shall show how I compared the values at the heart of the UK, Australian and Canadian healthcare systems.

# CHAPTER 4

# Using the model to analyse healthcare systems

## Background

The values underpinning any system should be clearly visible within the key policy documents governing the healthcare system in any country. It is worth noting that in the early 1990s the apparent cost of healthcare appeared to rise dramatically (*see* Figure 4.1).[17]

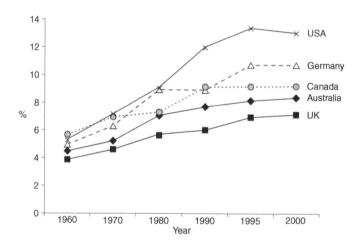

**Figure 4.1**  Total cost of healthcare expressed as % GDP.[17]

This rise and the overall upward trend were blamed on a number of factors, including:

• ageing population
• increasing cost of more sophisticated treatments
• increased expectations from consumers of healthcare.

This has been disputed by a range of authors in the years since: see, for example, Deber,[18] who points out that the cost of healthcare is measured as a percentage of gross domestic product (GDP), and in the early 1990s there was a global recession and GDP fell in many countries (*see* Figure 4.2).

Whatever the reality, the knee-jerk reaction of many governments was to instigate healthcare reforms to control costs. We shall use these reforms to examine the values

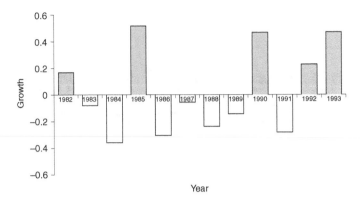

**Figure 4.2** Inflation adjusted growth in GDP (Canada 1982–1993).[19]

underpinning each system. The situation in the UK was perhaps a little different, with cost-cutting healthcare reforms introduced earlier by the Thatcher government from 1986 onwards. However, in this case, after 18 years a change in government in May 1997 led to a second wave of reform which we shall use for our comparison.

## Discerning values

In the three countries examined, policy reform was represented in a key document. The documents from the UK, Australia and Canada were respectively:

- *The New NHS*, Government White Paper, 1997[15]
- *Report to Parliament of the Senate Committee on Hospitals*, 2000[20]
- *Final Report of the National Forum on Health*, 1998.[21]

In addition, in each country, quality assurance documents were produced to describe how these values were to be put into practice. Therefore, a corresponding document in each country was considered to ensure that the values represented in the policy documents were the same as those against which operational performance was measured. The three documents used for this analysis were:

- *A First-class Service*, Department of Health, 1998[22]
- *Final Report of the National Expert Advisory Group on Safety and Quality in Australian Healthcare*, 1999[23]
- *Quest for Quality in Canadian Health Care*, Health Canada, 2000.[24]

Whilst the documents may not have been written specifically to measure how well the stated values were put into practice, they should reflect the operational realities prevailing in the countries at the time.

A qualitative approach was designed to discern the values present in the documents. The themes emerging from the documents were first considered and then classified according to a framework adapted from the work of Garvin.[25]

# Our classification framework for values

Garvin was concerned with the deceptively complex question of 'what does quality mean?', which in the context of healthcare could be viewed as the purpose of this book, although the 'q word' has I think been devalued in the time since Garvin's work. He proposed a multi-perspective model of quality, based upon five 'views' (*see* Table 4.1).

**Table 4.1**   Summary of Garvin's views of quality[25]

| View | Meaning |
| --- | --- |
| Transcendent | Absolute excellence |
| Product-based | Higher quality means higher cost |
| User-based | Fitness for purpose |
| Manufacturing | Conformance to specification |
| Value-based | Quality at a specific price |

We shall now consider his views in more detail, and specifically examine what they mean within the context of healthcare.

## The transcendent view

This view relates quality to innate excellence. Another word for this might be 'elegance'. This is the classical definition of quality, in tune with the *Oxford English Dictionary*. It is impossible to quantify and is difficult to apply in a meaningful sense to healthcare. An attempt to build in a high degree of innate excellence to healthcare is likely to be constrained by resources. Seeking to build healthcare along these lines is inevitably expensive, and thus resource constraints will tend to emphasise the value-based view, described below, rather than the transcendent view.

## The product-based view

This view is the economist's view: the higher the quality, the higher the cost. The basis for this view is that it costs money to provide higher quality. This is a commonly held view about healthcare. Better care and quicker access to services are commonly linked to more doctors, nurses and hospital beds. However, in certain areas better practice may also be cheaper. Examples of this may be found in screening programmes where health screening, e.g. for blood pressure, cervical cancer and child immunisation, can actually save money in the long term by keeping people healthy rather than treating people when they get ill. Also, the growing practice of clinical audit is highlighting areas where practice can be improved without necessarily increasing costs.

   This is the classic 'quality is free' argument, proposed by the likes of Crosby,[26] translated from manufacturing to healthcare. Crosby argues that by changing practice and reducing wastage, savings can be achieved in manufacturing which outweigh the costs of setting up new procedures.

However, unfortunately, this is by no means universal. Many improved practices will involve new technology, requiring investment. Once wastage is removed, improvements in waiting lists can only be achieved by more resources.

Many of the screening programmes, which are cost-effective in the long term, are expensive in the short term. For example, the growth in screening programmes in the UK has driven up computerisation rates amongst family doctors from around 25% to 90%. This represents a major investment where the cost must be set against the savings as illness is reduced.

Further, if screening programmes are justified on cost grounds alone, then programmes advantageous to health but less advantageous on cost grounds may be marginalised, e.g. breast cancer screening. Some people have also questioned the health benefits of such programmes, for example Charles Wright in Canada.[14]

From a health perspective, it is still better to prevent illness rather than treat it, and screening programmes in this category that are clinically effective but not cost-effective are good examples of Garvin's product-based view, i.e. higher quality of care costs more.

This view is often most pronounced in countries with strong private healthcare systems and/or a high technology infrastructure, e.g. the USA, and in the rest of the book we shall refer to it as the resource-based view, as healthcare is a service, not a product.

## The user-based view

This view was first championed in the 1940s, and is traditionally expressed as fitness for purpose. It is sometimes represented as patient satisfaction. This can, however, be a simplification.

Fitness for purpose implies that the service provided meets the needs of patients. Thus, it certainly includes aspects of performance such as waiting times, access to services and patient satisfaction. However, overall fitness for purpose is compromised if waiting times are reduced by emphasising the treatment of conditions that are quick, easy and cheap at the expense of more seriously ill patients.

It is also compromised if waiting times are reduced at the expense of reducing the effectiveness of treatment provided, leading to an increase in readmissions. Many measures currently applied to the UK NHS which purport to measure NHS fitness for purpose, e.g. waiting times, waiting list sizes and number of patients treated, actually measure the quantity of healthcare provided rather than the quality.

It is strong in systems that place an emphasis upon quality of life and take a holistic view of patient care, and place a priority upon integrated care including integrated social and home care. We shall therefore in the context of healthcare refer to it as the patient-based view.

## The manufacturing view

The manufacturer's view measures quality in terms of conformance to requirements. A simple example might be the dimensions of a component. The specification will state both the required dimension and the tolerance that will be acceptable.

The manufacturing view emerges in healthcare in a number of ways. The first is the introduction of protocols and standards for specific clinical procedures. These may be regarded as a specification for a clinical procedure. In the UK, one of the stated outcomes of the clinical audit process is the introduction of standards to disseminate 'best practice'.

However, the setting of such standards is by no means universal and in practice it is rarely possible to provide guidelines that embody 'best practice'. Guidelines will prevent bad practice and can lead to uniform improvements where existing practice is flawed. However, best practice generally requires skills and judgement, which are not easily enshrined in deterministic procedures. Thus the result of guidelines can be problem avoidance rather than promotion of excellence.

Much has been written on the lack of good evidence to support guidelines in many areas of healthcare. For example, in 1985, the United States Congressional Office of Technology Assessment estimated that only 10–20% of clinical practice was supported by randomised controlled trials.[27] In 1991, there was an estimate that as few as 15% of medical decisions were based on the results of rigorous evidence.[28] Another analysis that approached the topic from a different perspective suggested that just more than 50% of in-patient general medicine had level three evidence to support care provided in a hospital setting.[29]

These data suggest that a significant amount of clinical practice does not have an explicit evidence base. However, the extent of this is still being debated. This limits the effectiveness of tools such as clinical practice guidelines that have been developed to support clinicians in adopting evidence-based practices. James (1999)[28] estimates that only 10–20% of guideline steps are covered by any sort of published research.[30]

Best practice requires the exercising of judgement rather than following a deterministic procedure. This encourages doctors to view quality in terms of meeting a specification. If the specification is met, the doctor has fulfilled his obligation, even if the patients' aspirations are not met. The biggest threat to this lies in the increasing threat of malpractice suits.

This view is characterised by a range of systems which emphasise systems and process above all else, and therefore for our purposes we shall refer to it as the systemic view of healthcare.

## The value-based view

In a business context, this is the ability to provide what the customer requires at a price they can afford. In a public health service, the customer is ultimately the tax-paying public represented by the Government. A value-based view of quality assesses the cost-effectiveness of a service or treatment.

The value-based view is not generally made explicit in healthcare as it is usually politically unacceptable for politicians to admit that healthcare budgets are finite. However, as has been noted, in the early 1990s, during an economic recession, the percentage of GDP spent on healthcare in many countries rose sharply, leading to a much more public debate on the cost of providing healthcare.

This view is characterised by an emphasis upon the cost of healthcare and upon analyses based upon economic rather than health outcomes. However, value is a virtue required of any healthcare system, and therefore we shall retain the terminology for our analysis.

# A framework of values

In order to construct the framework to evaluate our policy document, we shall make two assumptions:

- The transcendent view of quality represents an overall view of quality, in essence a combination of the other views.
- The other views of quality may, and often do, conflict with each other.

It follows from these assumptions that the transcendent view represents the optimum balance between these different views.

In applying Garvin's views[25] to the values underpinning healthcare policy, we are recognising that ultimately those values determine the priorities that we wish to set within our healthcare policy. As such, we are seeking an optimum balance of priorities based upon our values, rather than a transcendent level of excellence.

In human terms, we must decide whether to focus on providing Harold's hip replacement more quickly and effectively or on putting in place medical resources which may never be needed to deal with any emergency that arises in Daphne's childbirth.

In order to explore the values present in our documents, we go through a three-step process:

1 Identify the values which form themes within the documents.
2 Characterise them as representing one of our four views of quality.
3 Identify the transcendent view of quality expressed within the document as the totality of the values in the document, recognising their inherent conflicts.

However, to define a representation of the balance of values underpinning our health policy, we need to define the relationships between the views represented within the document. In order to do this we need a representation that provides for interactions between all four views. Therefore we will set the four views of quality as the corners of a tetrahedron (*see* Figure 4.3).

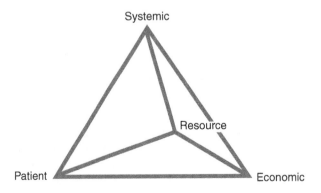

**Figure 4.3**   The schematic tetrahedral representation of optimising policy values.

A policy document based upon only one type of the values would be represented as sitting at one of the points of the tetrahedron (*see* Figure 4.4).

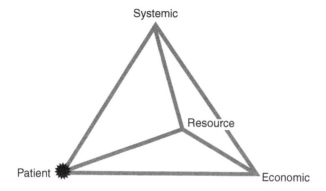

**Figure 4.4**   This policy document is based only upon patient-based values.

One based upon two types of values occupies a point on the edge of the tetrahedron (*see* Figure 4.5).

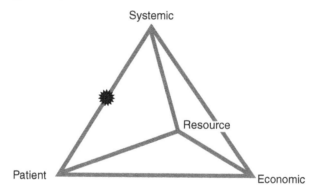

**Figure 4.5**   This policy document is based only upon patient- and systemic-based values.

One based upon three types of values occupies a point on a face of the tetrahedron (*see* Figure 4.6).

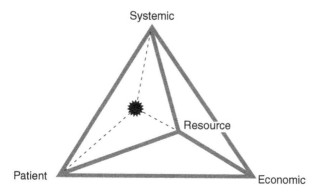

**Figure 4.6**   This policy document is based upon patient-, resource- and systemic-based values.

A policy which balances all four types of values occupies a point within the tetrahedron. I shall not attempt to draw one of these at present!

# Discerning drivers

Our overall model recognises that whilst policy is based upon values, it is then influenced by other factors, which we have called drivers. Once we have established the values present in the initial policy documents and the accompanying quality assurance documents, we shall use interviews carried out in the three countries to establish where operational practice is actually headed. From this we should be able to establish what the key drivers actually are.

# CHAPTER 5

# Values underpinning policy development

## The UK

*The New NHS* White Paper[15] was introduced to establish the basis of the NHS for the next ten years. In practice, quality is one of the major themes of the document:

> A National Health Service which offers people prompt, high-**quality** treatment and care when and where they need it.
>
> (para 1.1)

> In order to sustain the NHS, while making it both modern and dependable, this White Paper proposes a new drive for **quality**.
>
> (para 1.22)

> Patients will be guaranteed national standards of excellence so that they can have confidence in the **quality** of the services they receive.
>
> (para 1.4)

Within the theme of quality, which permeates the whole document, there are two key sub-themes of standards and efficiency.

Standards emerge in a number of different guises: standards, indicators, National Service Frameworks and guidelines:

> The new NHS Charter will tell people about the **standards** of treatment and care they can expect of the NHS.
>
> (para 4.20)

> In order to achieve primary care trust status, primary care groups will need to demonstrate that they have a systematic approach to monitoring and developing clinical **standards** in practices.
>
> (para 5.34)

> The NHS Executive is working with the profession to develop **indicators** to assess the effectiveness of primary care at national and health authority level.
>
> (para 5.33)

> The Government will work with the professions and representatives of users and carers to establish clearer, evidence-based **National Service Frameworks** for major care areas and disease groups.
>
> (para 7.8)

> The Government will spread best practice and drive clinical and cost-effectiveness in a number of ways: ... by developing a programme of new evidence-based **National Service Frameworks** setting out the patterns and levels of service which should be provided for patients with certain conditions ... by establishing a new National Institute for Clinical Excellence which will promote clinical and cost-effectiveness by producing **clinical guidelines** and audits for dissemination throughout the NHS.
>
> (para 7.6)

At the same time, this is balanced by an emphasis upon efficiency, sometimes described as cost-effectiveness:

> There will be new incentives and new sanctions to improve **quality** and **efficiency**.
>
> (para 1.4)

> There will have to be big gains in **quality** and big gains in **efficiency** across the whole NHS.
>
> (para 1.24)

> But that extra money has to produce major gains in **quality** and **efficiency**.
>
> (para 2.24)

> **Efficiency** and **quality** should go hand in hand.
>
> (para 3.8)

> The Government is determined that the services and treatment that patients receive across the NHS should be based on the best evidence of what does and does not work and what provides best value for money (clinical and **cost-effectiveness**).
>
> (para 7.5)

In terms of our conceptual framework these themes are firmly within the systemic- and value-based views of quality (*see* Box 5.1).

The New NHS White Paper[15] in 1997 spawned a range of documents to describe how it would be implemented. The document describing the quality assurance arrangements was called *A First-class Service*, published by the Department of Health in 1998.[31]

This document was described in *Health Service Circular*, volume 113 as a 'consultation document on quality in the new NHS'. It has a different emphasis from the White Paper and more of an operational feel. It describes the role of key organisations, especially the National Institute for Clinical Excellence (NICE).

---

**Box 5.1** Principal value types represented within the UK *The New NHS* White Paper

*Resource-based*

*Patient-based*

*Systemic-based*
Standards:
• indicators
• National Service Frameworks (NSFs)
• guidelines

*Economic-based*
Efficiency
Resources
Costs
Cost-effectiveness

---

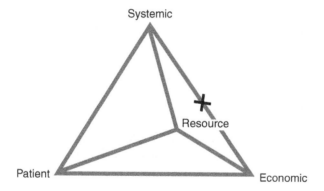

**Figure 5.1** Transcendent view of value types found in *The New NHS* White Paper.[15]

The themes emerging from the document are different from the White Paper. Quality is no longer linked to resources in such a significant way. There are a few links made between quality and efficiency:

> The Government will ensure there is accountability for both **efficiency** and **quality** throughout the NHS.
>
> (para 1.8)

but this forms a much more minor theme than in the White Paper. However, the role of NICE is strongly emphasised:

> A new **National Institute for Clinical Excellence (NICE),** promoting clinical and cost-effectiveness through guidance and audit, to support front-line staff.
>
> (para 2.6)

**NICE** will be responsible for appraisal and the production of guidance ... and its dissemination to the NHS.

(para 2.9)

Guidance from **NICE** will include guidelines for the management of certain diseases or conditions and guidance on the appropriate use of particular interventions.

(para 2.13)

The role of NICE emphasises the theme of standards as found in *The New NHS* White Paper, and standards are a recurring theme here too:

This Government wants to see a National Health Service which offers dependable, high **standards** of care and treatment everywhere.

(para 2.2)

The main elements are: clear national **standards** for services and treatments....

(para 5.1)

and this theme is emphasised again through the advocacy of NSFs, use of evidence and audit.

**National Service Frameworks (NSFs)** will:

- set national standards and define service models for a specific service or care group
- put in place programmes to support implementation
- establish performance measures against which progress within an agreed timescale will be measured.

(para 2.34)

**National Service Frameworks** will address the 'whole system of care'.

(para 2.38)

Such national guidance will mean that interventions with good **evidence** of clinical and cost-effectiveness will be actively promoted, so that patients have faster access to treatments known to work.

(para 2.17)

This can be done through clinical **audit**, which allows them to look at what they are doing against agreed standards and, where necessary, make changes to practice.

(para 2.18)

The other major theme running through this document is patients and meeting their needs and expectations:

High-quality care should be a right for every **patient** in the NHS.

(para 1.1)

Every **patient** judges the performance of the whole NHS by the quality of the care he or she receives in their local GP surgery, their local hospital, from their local midwife or health visitor, their local laboratory.

(para 1.5)

**Patients** experience the NHS as a local service and the needs of the East End of London are different from the needs of East Surrey.

(para 1.11)

And it is why the Government is setting such store on the views of **patients** acting as a positive lever for change.

(para 1.29)

The high-quality care that **patients** have a right to **expect**.

(para 4.1)

In terms of our conceptual framework these themes are firmly within the systemic- and value-based views of quality (*see* Box 5.2).

---

**Box 5.2**  Principal value types represented within the UK document *A First-class Service*[31]

| | |
|---|---|
| *Resource-based* | *Systemic-based* |
| | Standards |
| | NICE |
| | NSFs |
| | Evidence |
| | Audit |
| | |
| *Patient-based* | *Economic-based* |
| Patient expectations | Cost-effectiveness |

---

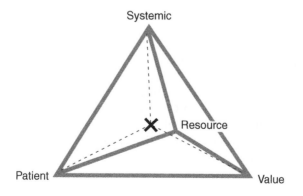

**Figure 5.2**  Transcendent view of value types found in the document *A First-class Service*.[31]

However, some of the reality has indicated that the emphasis upon cost-effectiveness remains. For example, the most controversial advice from NICE has not proved to be around clinical effectiveness, but around cost-effectiveness, with refusals to endorse treatments for influenza and multiple sclerosis, amongst others, on cost grounds.

# Australia

The introduction to the *Report to Parliament of the Senate Committee on Hospitals*[20] lays out the background:

> In July 1999, following widespread public concern about the state of the public hospital system, State Premiers and Territory Chief Ministers called on the Federal Government to establish an independent inquiry, preferably to be conducted by the Productivity Commission, into the health system. In response to the request, the Federal Government stated that it did not believe such a review would be productive.
>
> (para 1.1)

> However, the Senate subsequently agreed to establish an inquiry and on 11 August 1999 the matter was referred to the Committee for inquiry and report by 30 June 2000.
>
> (para 1.2)

Although Chapter 7 of the report is explicitly about quality assurance, the entire report is in reality concerned with the quality of the hospital service.

This report takes a predominantly resource-centred view of quality. This reflects the background of the Committee as much as the terms of reference of the report itself.

The key themes of this document are:

- funding
- the role of the private sector
- equity of access
- reporting systems.

The issue of funding is a major theme of the entire document:

> The foregoing discussion encapsulates a dilemma evident in the evidence on **funding** issues received by the Committee in this inquiry. Some participants have argued that Australia is spending about the right amount on health at 8.5 per cent of GDP. However, the majority of submissions regard the level of funding for public hospitals to be inadequate.
>
> (para 2.6)

The report also argues that funding increases must be matched by evidence of quality improvement:

> **Quality** improvements will remain an 'optional extra' in our health sys-
> tem until new **funding** arrangements are developed and implemented
> that require specific quality measures to be built into the entire system.
>
> (para 7.51)

and for the need for indicators to measure effectiveness and efficiency:

> As noted earlier in the chapter, in NSW the Government has developed
> a performance measurement framework for area health services that
> encompass indicators such as **effectiveness**, **efficiency**, safety and
> access.
>
> (para 7.128)

The report notes concern over the increasing demand placed upon healthcare and the funding implications:

> By contrast, the ability of governments to continue increasing health
> expenditure to meet **demand** is limited by finite budgets. These three
> factors – ageing of the population, advances in medical technology and
> expectations of consumers – are those most commonly advanced to
> explain increasing health expenditure in developed countries. The ageing
> of the population has received much attention and some dire predic-
> tions have been made of its possible future effect on Australia's health
> expenditure.
>
> (para 2.16)

> This rate of increase is not sufficient to meet the **demand** on public
> hospitals.
>
> (para 2.29)

Partly in response to these concerns, one of the major themes of the report is the exploration of the role of the private sector, and particularly its relationship to the funding question:

> The private sector has expanded in all states and, as the Productivity
> Commission has stated, governments have sought increasingly to involve
> the private sector with the provision of healthcare. Factors contributing
> to this include (self-imposed) funding constraints on governments which
> have limited their capacity to invest in new, or to expand existing, public
> hospital facilities and the perception that there would be cost savings
> and improvements in quality of care through greater private sector
> involvement.
>
> (para 6.28)

Until the late 1970s, many private for-profit hospitals were small, often owned and run by medical practitioners. However, developments over recent times have seen an expansion of the operation of private for-profit operators with corporations entering the market.

(para 6.1)

The link is made between private healthcare and the provision of high-technology services:

> In relation to the type of service provided, two studies were noted. The first, by Professor J Richardson and I Robertson, studied the likelihood of patients receiving a costly **hi-tech procedure** after hospitalisation with an acute myocardial infarction (AMI). It was found that those in private care were, at the end of eight weeks, 100 to 400 per cent more likely to receive a high-technology, high-cost procedure (angiography or a revascularisation) than patients treated in public hospitals. After 12 months a 100 per cent differential was preserved.
>
> (para 6.44)

However, this paragraph is followed by the following observation about the *quality* of care:

> Professor Richardson stated that there was no indication of differences in **quality** of life from the study (or whether these results suggest over servicing in the private sector, or under servicing in the public sector or a mix of both). However, 'if there is no difference there then that simply means we are doing more [in the private sector] for the same outcomes. That is costly.'
>
> (para 6.45)

The report goes on to highlight the greater costs of private care, even for the public system:

> The study found that private expenditures significantly exceeded public costs and 'perversely, because of the public reimbursement of medical and pharmaceutical costs, generated **higher costs for public Medicare** than if the patient had been admitted to the public hospital.'
>
> (para 6.47)

A sub-theme emerging in the debate about the public–private mix is access to care, where the report argues that the increased use of the private sector leads to reduced access for vulnerable groups:

> The changes to the level of service provision have significant implications for **access to care**. This is particularly so when the hospital in question is the only provider for the region. This is the case for the Latrobe Hospital which replaced two public hospitals that were closed at Moe and Taralgon.
>
> (para 6.69)

A further matter raised in relation to **access to quality care** concerned the changes in the public health sector workforce. Concerns were expressed that the supply of specialist medical staff in public hospitals may decline as a result of co-locations and expansion of the use of private hospitals. It was argued that this might lead to fewer specialists available to provide services in the public sector and thereby impact adversely on public sector waiting lists.

The increased reliance on part-time and casual hospital staff was also noted as an outcome of recent changes. It was argued that this increased pressures on staff and was detrimental to the **quality of care**.

(para 6.70)

However, this theme of equity of access also emerges in relation to rural healthcare:

People living in **rural and remote areas** also have less access to healthcare compared to their metropolitan counterparts.

(para 2.19)

The final major theme running through this report is the need for better information and reporting systems. Three types of reporting are highlighted:

- financial
- effectiveness
- adverse incidents.

The report notes the need to improve financial transparency and to take a more holistic view of costs:

The emphasis of this financial reporting should be on transparency rather than obfuscation, which characterises much of the reporting at present.

(para 2.45, recommendation 10)

The right question is not how much money is going to hospitals in rural areas but how much money is going to health services in rural areas.

(para 2.7)

The report calls for better reporting of clinical effectiveness, and incentivised funding noted above to support this:

The most commonly identified deficiency was gaps in the types of data collected. These gaps included data on health outcomes, **effectiveness** and cost-effectiveness of services.

(para 8.2)

A sub-theme was a call for the better use of existing data:

We do in Australia have an extraordinarily good database by world standards, but we do not use it. Through the linkage of records we could make an enormous impact onto this pool of ignorance about the effectiveness of different services.

(para 8.20)

Notwithstanding this and other supporting comments, the report highlights the need for electronic health records with a view to providing better information and facilitating better reporting:

A view was expressed in many submissions that data collection to date has tended to focus on costs and payment systems at the expense of other areas.

(para 8.3)

That funding for patient care and funding for data collection and perform- ance measurement should be separately and transparently identified and acquitted. Sufficient staff should be employed in public hospitals to ensure that both functions are undertaken effectively.

(Recommendation 40)

That the urgent development of adequate IT [information technology] systems in the health sector be undertaken, especially in relation to integrated management systems within hospitals and integrated patient records.

(Recommendation 41)

That the Commonwealth and the States commit the necessary resources to implement the HealthConnect proposal.

(Recommendation 42)

The third part of the report's recommendations on better reporting was the call for better reporting of adverse events:

There is little data on **adverse events** in Australia.

(para 7.6)

This report is large and wide-ranging. It is not surprising to find that there is a wide range of quality perspectives represented. In terms of our conceptual framework these themes may be seen to represent all four views of quality within the con- ceptual framework (*see* Box 5.3).

The National Expert Advisory Group on Safety and Quality in Australian Health- care reported at the request of Australian health ministers on quality matters within the Australian system. The Group was asked to:

identify those safety and quality matters that would benefit from national effort and coordination.

(Executive summary, para 2)

**Box 5.3** Principal value types represented within the Australian Report to Parliament of the Senate Committee on Hospitals[20]

*Resource-based*
Private sector
New technology
Increased demand
Funding constraints

*Patient-based*
Patients
Equity of access

*Systemic-based*
Adverse events reporting
Evidence-based practice
Information

*Economic-based*
Funding
Cost
Efficiency
Demand

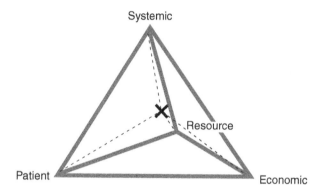

**Figure 5.3** Transcendent view of value types found in the *Australian Report to Parliament of the Senate Committee on Hospitals*.[20]

The methodology is described in the next paragraph:

> In considering this matter, the Expert Group reviewed past studies and reports and 115 public submissions, and met with a wide range of stakeholders and experts throughout Australia and overseas. As a result of this process, the Expert Group believes that the actions identified by the Taskforce on Quality in Australian Healthcare (1996) and in the Expert Group's Interim Report (1998) need to be implemented at all levels of the health system and in all healthcare agencies and organisations, public and private, to address the system-wide matters that could improve the safety and quality of healthcare in Australia.
>
> (Executive summary, para 3)

The resulting document has two main themes. The first is the need for systems and a systemic approach. This is complemented by recognising the needs of consumers, although the report does refer to patients explicitly in a number of places. There is a major sub-theme around the mechanisms to deliver the required systems.

The systemic approach is highlighted by many references throughout the report:

> That health ministers establish an Australian Council for Safety and Quality in Healthcare to facilitate national actions in those areas outlined in Recommendation 2 to improve safety and quality in healthcare through:
>
> - ...
> - promoting a **systemic approach** to safety and quality within the healthcare system and within the community at large.
>
> (Recommendation 3)

The report argues that a systemic approach is required to address systemic problems:

> - There is a need for reform within the Australian health system to reduce fragmentation, improve information sharing processes and coordinate action to address **systemic safety and quality problems** across all sectors and within and between the public and private healthcare environments.
>
> (Key point, p.17)

The report has a major sub-theme concerned with the mechanisms required to implement this systemic approach, including accreditation, adverse event reporting, information and evidence-based practice:

> The majority of submissions supported the need for some form of external review of healthcare organisations, including **accreditation** processes, to be strongly encouraged by State and Territory Governments.
>
> (p.27)

> - Development of best practice guidelines to support legislation to enable the appropriate and timely investigation of incidents, 'near misses' and **adverse events**.
>
> (p.38)

> In order to support better frameworks for quality management, **information** systems are required to enable the flow of patient **information** within organisations and across healthcare services, and to support the evaluation of health service safety and quality.
>
> (p.29)

> The Expert Group considers that a quality Australian health system would be one in which **evidence-based practice** is in day-to-day use with the infrastructure to support it.
>
> (p.15)

The complementary theme is that of consumers and patients as consumers:

> - **Consumer** feedback and participation, including complaints, are an important part of systemic lessons and quality improvement.
>
> (p.15)

- An integrated national agenda in pursuit of a quality health system must address safety and quality across a number of sectors in relation to individual consumers, vulnerable and at-risk populations and the system as a whole.

- It is important that health administrators and providers embed safety and quality improvement into their role in providing patient care and therefore focus more explicitly on the outcomes for consumers.

(Key points, p.16)

Once again, information is a key sub-theme as a mechanism for achieving consumer participation with provision of information for consumers identified as a priority area for research funding:

> ... undertaking studies into quality improvement approaches in the health system which could be applied nationally, e.g. research to identify effective methods for provision of health information to consumers.

> ... disseminating results of research and identified good practice in each action area to healthcare organisations, providers and consumers, e.g. identified effective and non-effective models of consumer participation, evidence-based practice, information flows, investigations into incidents and adverse events, performance measurement and curricula for education and training of health providers.

(pp.37–8)

In terms of our conceptual framework these themes are firmly within the systemic- and value-based views of quality (*see* Box 5.4).

---

**Box 5.4**   Principal value types represented within the Australian Report to Parliament of the Senate Committee on Hospitals[20]

| *Resource-based* | *Systemic-based* |
|---|---|
| | Systemic approach |
| | Adverse events |
| | Evidence-based practice |
| | Accreditation |
| | Information |
| *Patient-based* | *Economic-based* |
| Consumers | |
| Patients | |
| Information | |
| Dissemination | |

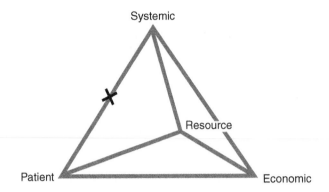

**Figure 5.4** Transcendent view of value types found in the final report of the National Expert Advisory Group on Safety and Quality in Australian Healthcare.[20]

# Canada[32]

The National Forum on Health was an extended consultation process carried out in Canada.[21] This document is the final report on a process that commissioned research and took opinions from many groups. It is perhaps more explicit in its expression of values and beliefs than any of the other documents. As such, three major themes emerge:

- preserving and extending the principles and practice of the Canada Health Act
- recommendations will depend upon resources
- amount and pace of change.

The theme of preserving and extending the principles and practice of the Canada Health Act is the most important of this report:

> The Forum recommends the following as the key features that must be preserved and protected:
>
> - public funding for medically necessary services
> - the 'single payer' model
> - the five principles of the **Canada Health Act**
> - a strong federal/provincial/territorial partnership.

In practice, the five principles of the Canada Health Act become the sub-themes within this theme:

> universality, accessibility, comprehensiveness, portability and public administration

and these principles are held to be inviolate.

However, there is recognition of the need for reform to provide adequate resources for both the preservation of existing services and the envisaged expansion:

> Preserving Medicare, however, also means **adapting to new realities** by:
>
> - expanding publicly funded services to include all medically neces-sary services and, in the first instance, home care and drugs
> - **reforming** primary care funding, organization and delivery.

This theme of adequate resourcing is explored throughout the text:

> Because of the magnitude of drug expenditures, increasing the share of public **funding** will hinge on the availability of fiscal resources.

> While we recognize that implementing our recommendations concern-ing children would require significant additional **funding**, we have set them out in order of priority and believe that they can be implemented over time as fiscal circumstances permit.

The tone of the presentation of the funding theme is different from that in the UK and Australian documents which often seem to present cost-efficiency as an end in itself. In this report, whilst there is recognition of economic reality and the need to prioritise objectives, there is an assertion that in order to meet the key health priorities, resources must be found:

> Regardless of which **funding** methods are chosen, there should be safeguards to ensure that high-quality care continues to be provided to those whose conditions incur higher costs.

And the argument is made, which is also found in the Australian hospitals report, that not finding the money through the public system will ultimately lead to greater costs:

> Our recommendations require action now, but some actions can be taken in small steps as fiscal circumstances permit. Implementing many of our recommendations would in fact entail a reshuffling of existing spending from one source to another. In other cases, we have recom-mended initiatives that are costly, but we have done so only because the alternatives – doing nothing or doing too little – will in the end **cost even more**.

> If we focus on total costs and value for money, the evidence suggests that increasing the scope of public expenditure may be the key to **reducing total costs**.

> We believe that implementing our recommendations on pharmaceuticals will, in the long run, result in a net **decrease in total drug costs** for Canadians.

This is also linked to the third theme, which is the recognition of the need to control the amount and rate of change. One sub-theme within this is the need to match fiscal circumstances, as described above. However, there is also the recognition, notably absent from the UK policy documents, that there is a need to implement evolutionary rather than revolutionary change:

> Rapid change always raises concerns.

> However, because we are not starting with a blank slate, we must be careful about the pace of change so that both the public and the health-care providers maintain their confidence in the system – a difficult balancing act.

However, this may be a little disingenuous, since the report is explicit in its support for the existing value framework of the healthcare system. Contrast this with the UK where the White Paper[15] details the shortcomings of the existing system.

In terms of our conceptual framework these themes are firmly within the patient- and value-based views of quality, although the patient-based view is given clear precedence in the report (*see* Box 5.5).

---

**Box 5.5**   Principal value types represented within the Final Report of the National Forum on Health (Canada)[21]

*Resource-based*                                              *Systemic-based*

*Patient-based*                                               *Economic-based*
Canada Health Act:                                           Resources
- universality                                               Need for reform
- accessibility
- comprehensiveness
- portability
- public administration

---

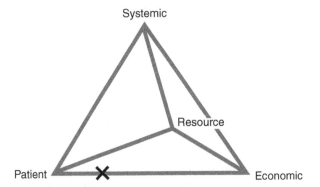

**Figure 5.5**   Transcendent view of value types found in the final report of the National Forum on Health (Canada).[21]

This places the transcendent view of quality on the patient-value edge of our conceptual tetrahedron, nearer the patient end than the value end (*see* Figure 5.5).

The *Quest for Quality in Canadian Healthcare* document[24] has two major themes. The first is the use of continuous quality improvement (CQI) as the means to achieving better quality of care. Within this there is an emphasis upon the following sub-themes as the means to achieve this:

- process
- planning
- measurement and indicators.

The second theme is the need to take account of the needs of all the stakeholders. This includes patients and also the clinicians and other staff delivering care and the wider community. Within this theme there are the sub-themes of team-building and education.

The advocacy of CQI as the mechanism for quality improvement is very strong and runs throughout the document:

> **Continuous quality improvement** is a management philosophy that offers promise to save our system through the reduction of inefficiencies and inappropriate variation as identified by line healthcare professionals and support staff.
>
> (p.11)

This advocacy is reinforced by the sub-themes running through the document, which represent the means to achieve improvement.

The first is an emphasis upon process:

> The next step is to identify key **processes** for improvement.
>
> (p.100)

> Key processes: **processes** key to the organization's mission are described and documented. Those responsible for each **process** are identified. This exercise will enable the organization to assess its process capabilities, and will provide a baseline from which to choose **processes** to review and improve.
>
> (p.118)

The second sub-theme concerned with the implementation of CQI is planning:

> Quality in **planning** can prevent many of the problems within the organization and with customers that occur in staffing, capital expenditure and integration.
>
> (p.17)

> Strategy development becomes an interactive process of **planning**, taking leveraged actions and learning from success and failure.
>
> (p.80)

Measurement and the appropriate use of indicators is the third major sub-theme concerned with the implementation of CQI:

> **Measurement** tells us whether innovations should be kept, changed or rejected to understand causes and to clarify aims.
>
> (p.58)

> Successful improvement requires facility in the **measurement** of progress toward aims, of the needs and status of patients and other consumers of care, and of local process characteristics that may be related to aims (Nelson *et al.* 1998).
>
> (cited on p.62)

> **Indicators** should actually measure what they are intended to (validity); they should provide the same answer if measured by different people in similar circumstances (reliability); they should be able to measure change (sensitivity); and they should reflect changes only in the situation concerned. In reality, these criteria are difficult to achieve, and indicators, at best, are indirect or partial measures of a complex situation.
>
> (cited on p.155)

> Work is needed in each area of **indicator** development.
>
> (p.157)

The presentation of this sub-theme in this document clearly recognises the complexity of the issue.

The second major theme is one of taking into account the needs of all the stakeholders, including the need for education, learning and teamwork. Whilst this is presented as part of the implementation of CQI, it is significant enough to be a major theme in its own right:

> Quality in healthcare can be reflected through the perspectives of its different **stakeholders**: the patient (client, resident), the provider, the funder and society.
>
> (p.13)

> These criteria must take into account the values and interests of the decision makers, the implementers, the organization and the broader **stakeholders**.
>
> (p.84)

The need for education is a major sub-theme:

> Appropriate **education** for all involved in quality management is a priority.
>
> (p.16)

And the need for organisational learning, as distinct from education, is also emphasised:

> The organization of the future requires a culture where ... **learning** is a constant.
>
> (p.69)

> Innovation and **learning** are the most challenging areas in which to develop measures; these measures are important since they assess organizational capacity for improvement and change.
>
> (p.189)

The final sub-theme in this area is teamwork:

> By pooling their skills, talents and knowledge, the **team** can tackle complex and chronic problems and develop effective solutions through mutual understanding of the entire process.
>
> (p.90)

> Appropriately developed, trained **teams** can enable an organization to significantly improve the processes by which care and service are delivered.
>
> (p.90)

However, in recognising these sub-themes as belonging to a common theme, it should be recognised that the document ultimately identifies this entire theme as a means to an end, where the end is the provision of care to the patient or client:

> Success can only be achieved if all stakeholders in the provision of care focus first and foremost on the **client**.
>
> (cited on p.35)

In terms of our conceptual framework these themes are firmly within the systemic- and value-based views of quality (*see* Box 5.6).

---

**Box 5.6**  Principal value types represented within the *The Quest for Quality in Canadian Healthcare* document[24]

| | |
|---|---|
| *Resource-based* | *Systemic-based* |
| | CQI |
| | Process |
| | Planning |
| | Measurement and indicators |
| | |
| *Patient-based* | *Economic-based* |
| Stakeholders | |
| Education | |
| Learning | |
| Teamworking | |
| Client focus | |

---

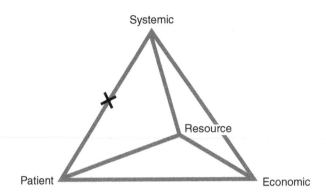

**Figure 5.6** Transcendent view of value types found in *The Quest for Quality in Canadian Healthcare* document.[24]

This places the transcendent view of quality on the systemic-patient edge of our conceptual tetrahedron (*see* Figure 5.6).

## Conclusions

In this chapter we have discerned the underlying values set out in key policy documents in our three comparator countries. The result indicates significant differences in the emphases within each system:

- The UK White Paper[15] emphasises the systemic view and the economic view.
- The Australian Report[20] represents all points of view and gives little clue as to emphasis, although the quality document focuses upon systemic and value-based aspects.
- The Canadian Forum Report[21] emphasises patients but recognises the need for economic constraints to be acknowledged.

In the following chapters we shall consider each country in more detail and consider whether the values underpinning policy have been driven off course by other factors, and indeed whether there is commitment to put policy objectives into practice.

# CHAPTER 6

# What is the reality in the UK?

## Historical development

Early advances in health in the UK* came about not as a result of healthcare, but as a result of improvements in housing and social conditions in the nineteenth century. Most significant was the provision of clean water for the growing urban centres where the engineering expertise of the Victorians was put to excellent use in both the building of reservoirs and the accompanying infrastructure, and the provision of an effective sewerage system.

Between the wars there was an increasing awareness of the social inequalities in healthcare provision, and the inability of the poor to pay for healthcare. The system was a private one. Some support was provided: for example, access to a doctor was free to the lower paid workers, but not their wives or children, but many slightly higher paid workers could not afford medical services. Hospitals charged for services, although some reimbursement schemes existed, but many could not afford to pay in the first place.

In practice, medical services for the poor were largely dependent upon charity, either that of philanthropists who set up schemes or that of individual doctors who provided some services *pro bono publico*.

Following the Second World War, the post-war Government brought in a range of reforms that included the 1944 Education Act as well as legislation to establish a National Health Service built upon the principle of being free at the point of delivery. The UK NHS was established in 1948.[33] The National Health Service became reality on 5 July 1948 in an atmosphere of post-war austerity, and health-care competed for scarce resources with other key areas, especially rehousing, which was the responsibility of the same Government minister as health.

The NHS brought a wide variety of health services together for the first time: hospital services, family practitioner services (doctors, pharmacists, opticians and dentists) and community-based services. The integration of the NHS has always been a problem, and remains one to this day.

The NHS was established with the principle of being free at the point of delivery of care. The combination of universality and a growing expectation together with an increasing range of treatments, e.g. cardiac surgery, hip replacements, quickly raised costs. However, even at this stage, some of this cost was offset by cheaper and better treatments. For example, improvements in the treatment of tuberculosis allowed hospital wards to be closed or diverted to other uses. There are interesting

---

* Much of the discussion that follows relates to England and not to the UK. This is not intended as a slur on the Celtic nations. A discussion of the differences between the home countries within the UK may be found on the website.

parallels in the concerns over the increasing costs of asthma drugs in the late 1990s, which are more than offset by the reductions in cost of emergency admissions.

In spite of such positive steps, costs continued to rise. Within three years of its creation, the NHS was forced to introduce some fees. Prescription charges were permitted by legislation in 1949 and introduced in 1952. A flat fee for ordinary dental treatment was brought in at the same time. Once again, many people looking back to the halcyon days of a truly 'free' NHS rarely appreciate that it was technically free only for the first year of its existence and only free in practice for the first three years.

The foundation of the new service was the family doctor or general practitioner. In spite of this, the contractual arrangements for hospital doctors were considerably more favourable than their colleagues in general practice. At the time of writing, hospital consultants retain their favourable 1948 working conditions. The Government adopted a policy of divide and rule amongst the medical profession. In more recent times the GP contracts have been rewritten, notably in 1990[34] and again at the time of writing.

However, when the NHS was established, the one concession that was won by GPs was the ability to operate as independent contractors within the NHS. This has been retained to this day, but is under threat as never before.

Then, as now, the family doctor acted as gatekeeper to the rest of the NHS, referring patients where appropriate to hospitals or specialist treatment and prescribing medicines and drugs. The first time this was questioned was in the late 1990s when most GPs opted out of 24-hour cover, and NHSDirect and a range of other initiatives such as walk-in centres were introduced to provide alternative advice and access mechanisms.

Dental services consisted of check-ups and all necessary fillings and dentures. There was a school dental service and a special priority service for expectant and nursing mothers and young children that was organised by local authorities. Eye tests were provided by ophthalmic opticians on production of a GP referral note.

Within the local communities new community health centres were built with accommodation and equipment supplied from public funds to enable a range of primary care services, including GPs, dentists, health visitors and others, to work together. There were also specialist ear clinics at which patients could get an expert opinion and, if needed, a new hearing aid.

As the NHS developed, fragmentation was a recurring theme. In 1962 the Porritt report criticised the separation of the NHS into three parts – hospitals, general practice and local health authorities – and called for unification.

Also in the 1960s, the need for an overall management strategy was recognised and a ten-year plan for the NHS established. The 1960s were generally an optimistic decade in the UK and advances in healthcare fed this optimism. However, as the decade closed and moved into the 1970s, inflation rose and morale fell.

In an attempt to address this fall in morale, a Royal Commission was established to investigate the NHS, which reported in 1976. In spite of, or perhaps because of, continuing advances in healthcare technology and an increasing emphasis upon management, the NHS continued to get further into debt and waiting lists grew during the 1980s.

In 1980, just as the UK began a period of the most right-wing Government since the Second World War, a major review of health inequalities was published. It had been commissioned by the Government and chaired by Sir Douglas Black. The Black Report and its successors have been instrumental in keeping health inequalities at the forefront of the public health agenda.

A major wave of reforms was introduced in the late 1980s. The Government of the day, led by Margaret Thatcher, sought to bring market forces into the NHS with the introduction of the so-called internal market, outlined in the 1989 White Paper, *Working for Patients*, and made law as the NHS and Community Care Act 1990. Before this Act a single, complex bureaucracy ran all aspects of the NHS. After the establishment of the internal market, 'purchasers' (health authorities and some family doctors) were given budgets to buy healthcare from 'providers' (acute hospitals, organisations providing care for the mentally ill, people with learning disabilities and the elderly, and ambulance services).

In order to become a 'provider' in the internal market, health organisations became NHS trusts, independent organisations with their own managements, and crucially for both the supporters and detractors of the system, competing with each other.

In reality, for a market to operate, there must be significant spare capacity in the system and 'customers' must be able to exercise choice. Capacity, let alone spare capacity, was in short supply in the NHS. The transaction costs of costing every procedure proved hugely expensive and in practice was not a precise science.

The unreal nature of the system was illustrated by the fact that the providers reserved the right to go back to the purchasers for more money if they got their sums wrong! Further, much of the population could not realistically be served by more than one hospital.

The election of a new Government in May 1997 brought a new approach to the NHS. Pledging itself to abolition of the internal market, the new Government set out an approach which aimed to build on what had worked previously, but discarding what had failed. It was a political necessity for a new Labour Government to move away from the ideological basis of competition. However, just as it is not clear how market driven the NHS of 1990–97 really was, so it is difficult to establish how cooperative the 'new NHS' really is.

The official version is that:

> A new White Paper issued by the Department of Health, *The New NHS: modern, dependable*, put forward a 'third way' of running the service – based on partnership and driven by performance. The paper set out an approach which promised to 'go with the grain' of efforts by NHS staff to overcome obstacles within the internal market, building on the moves which had already taken place in the NHS to move away from outright competition to a more collaborative approach.

The White Paper[15] described this approach as 'a new model for a new century', based on six key principles:

- to renew the NHS as a genuinely national service, offering fair access to consistently high-quality, prompt and accessible services right across the country
- second, to make the delivery of healthcare against these new national standards a matter of local responsibility, with local doctors and nurses in the driving seat in shaping services

- third, to get the NHS to work in partnership, breaking down organisational barriers and forging stronger links with local authorities
- fourth, to drive efficiency through a more rigorous approach to performance, cutting bureaucracy to maximise every pound spent in the NHS for the care of patients
- fifth, to shift the focus onto quality of care so that excellence would be guaranteed to all patients, with quality the driving force for decision making at every level of the service
- sixth, to rebuild public confidence in the NHS as a public service, accountable to patients, open to the public and shaped by their views.

Already by 2002, the new cooperative culture is being overtaken by a more directive approach from the centre. For example, the cooperative and advisory primary care groups (PCGs) described in the 1997 *The New NHS* White Paper have been replaced by primary care trusts (PCTs) with a more managerial and directive approach. Whilst this was envisaged in the White Paper, it has happened more quickly than was intended, and the PCTs resemble the previous managing health authorities rather than the PCGs. An indication of this is the appointment of staff from these management organisations. Many chief executives of the new PCTs have been brought in from outside the NHS altogether. Much of this is being driven by the quality agenda.

# The current situation viewed from an international perspective

The UK differs from Canada and Australia in not having a federal/provincial or Commonwealth/State split. This is a significant difference in the organisation of healthcare. Since 1999, however, there have been National Assemblies in Scotland and Wales and the legislative assembly in Northern Ireland was also re-established as a consequence of the negotiations there between the concerned parties. Even before devolution, each nation was responsible for managing its healthcare system, but the principles and functioning were basically the same throughout the UK. It remains to be seen whether the systems will diverge. There is some evidence of this happening in Scotland.

The UK NHS remains one of the most centrally managed and financed healthcare systems in the world. The central Government is not only involved in the financing of health services but is also heavily involved in the management and delivery of services. The current Government, having emphasised local flexibility in much of its early policy work, appears now to be retrenching with significant national standards work. This contrasts sharply with Canada, Germany and Sweden where the responsibility for healthcare is shared between the different levels of government.

Responsibility for social care, such as long-term residential nursing care, is shared between local government, various social services departments and the NHS, which has led to a long-standing problem of poor coordination. This problem currently manifests itself in the promised delivery of integrated care supported by integrated computerised records. The Data Protection Commissioner has ruled against the sharing of patient information on confidentiality grounds.

All residents of the UK are eligible for healthcare coverage under the NHS. The NHS coverage is more comprehensive than Canadian Medicare as it covers physicians, hospitals, prescription drugs, dental care and optical services, although many of these attract patient co-payments, with exemptions for the elderly and the poor. However, as in Canada, and in contrast to Australia, there are no user charges for physician services in the UK and hospital and specialist services are provided free of charge.

In the case of prescription drugs, there is a flat charge for each prescription written on the NHS. However, about 60% of the population benefit from exemptions and around 80% of prescriptions are written for people who are exempt. Frequent users who are not eligible for exemption may pay an annual charge instead of individual charges.

Within the NHS, general dental services are subject to a considerable amount of co-payment, with individuals paying 80% of the cost of their treatment up to a maximum figure set by the Government to aid clarity. Here as well, certain groups such as children are exempt.

In terms of private healthcare insurance, the UK differs from Canada in allowing people to purchase private insurance that covers the same benefits as the NHS if these services are supplied by providers working outside of the NHS. Private insurance takes two main forms: employer-sponsored insurance (59% of the total) and individual insurance policies. In just under one-third of the company schemes employees meet all or part of the premium costs. In 1996 there were 25 private healthcare insurers offering coverage in the UK. Seven of these were non-profit, provident insurers while the remaining 18 were commercial insurers. Two large insurers (PPP Healthcare and British United Provident Association [BUPA]) cover more than two-thirds of those covered by private healthcare insurance. There is some degree of vertical integration in the private healthcare sector as several of the large insurers are also amongst the major owners of the 230 medical/surgical hospitals that comprise the independent sector.

One of the major reasons given by people who take private insurance is they want the peace of mind of being able to have elective operations for themselves or their families more quickly or at more convenient times than if they depend on the National Health Service. This is a major motivation in a system where waiting times generally are long compared to Canada or Australia.

However, since primary care is essentially public in the UK, most people's predominant experience is of the NHS and they only resort to private healthcare when they perceive the NHS to be inadequate, usually in terms of access to care.

Until 1990, NHS hospitals were state owned and operated by the NHS through its regional health authorities. The budget of each regional health authority was determined by the central Government by means of a weighted capitation formula based on the healthcare needs of the regional population. Each hospital's budget was then determined regionally through an administrative process involving negotiations between its management and the relevant regional health authority. Hospital specialists were salaried employees of the NHS (but were also permitted to operate a private practice in parallel to the NHS).

A major critique of such a system was that regional health authorities were contracting, or purchasing, services on behalf of their local populations, but at the same time they were running the local hospitals. Thus, they had a pronounced conflict of interest aimed at protecting those hospitals.

In 1991, under the reforms of the Thatcher Government, regional health authorities ceased to manage hospitals and became responsible, as purchasing organisations, for contracting with NHS hospitals and private providers to deliver the services required by their resident populations. Hospitals, for their part, were transformed into NHS trusts; that is, not-for-profit organisations within the NHS but outside the control of the regional health authorities.

The first 57 NHS trusts were established in 1991, and all healthcare was provided by NHS trusts by 1995. Over the same period, many family doctors were also given their own budgets with which to buy healthcare from NHS trusts in a scheme called GP fund-holding. However, there was much more opposition to reform amongst the GPs. Not all GPs joined this scheme and their budgets were still controlled by health authorities which bought healthcare 'in bulk' from NHS trusts. When fund-holding was abandoned in 1997, only approximately 50% of GPs were fund-holders, in spite of apparently significant benefits being offered.

The new Government in 1997 claimed that the patients of GP fund-holders were often able to obtain treatment more quickly than patients of non-fund-holders. This led to accusations of the NHS operating a two-tier system, contrary to the founding principles of the NHS of fair and equal access to healthcare for all. The challenge remains to this day to make the NHS more responsive to the specific needs of its patients whilst ensuring equality of access nationwide.

NHS trusts were expected to compete for contracts from their 'purchasers' – health authorities and general practitioners – for the provision of clinical services. Each trust was expected to generate income through service contracts with purchasers and had to meet centrally specified financial objectives such as making a 6% return on its capital assets. Payments to hospitals thus depended on the contract signed with the purchasers. Typically, contracts specified what services were to be provided and the terms on which they were to be supplied.

The incoming Labour Government made much of its commitment to abolish the internal market. However, they have not announced plans to radically change the status of acute NHS trusts and have in addition created trusts to manage primary care. Trusts remain independent organisations within the NHS. However, their relationship with the regional health authorities has shifted from the previous emphasis on competition and financial performance toward a collaborative approach to quality of care. Changes where they have come have been in the primary care sector.

Authorities such as the World Bank have praised the introduction of the purchaser/provider split in the UK. In reality, it was characterised by high transaction costs and was never implemented in the full sense.

Chris Ham, Director of the Health Services Management Centre, in his evidence to the Romanow Commission on Health Care in Canada[32] said:

> I would say 'internal market' was always a bit of a misnomer in our case. I would say it was a managed market and it turned out to be a heavily politically-managed market.... They did not actually implement the internal market as it was intended from the beginning, so in practice I would say there was not ever a great deal of competition between hospitals and other healthcare providers and to that extent the so-called internal market experiment was never tested in the way that was intended at the outset.

The new Government has done significantly more in reorganising the primary care sector. When the NHS was established, GPs were allowed to operate as independent contractors within the NHS. This is similar to the situation in Australia and Canada. They were also permitted the right to private practice alongside their NHS work, although very little primary medical care in the UK is private. Only 3% of GP consultations are estimated to be in the private sector. By contrast, dental services have moved substantially away from NHS provision to private care, particularly during the 1990s when there was little Government commitment to maintaining an NHS dental service.

At present, GPs retain their independent contractor status. They are not employees of the NHS, as many people interviewed in Canada or Australia suggested.

However, the autonomy of GPs in the UK has been gradually eroded. First the provision of care by GPs was brought into a 'rostering system', requiring patients to register with one GP who then acted as a 'gatekeeper' to the rest of the healthcare system. Patients could only be admitted to hospital, see a specialist or have their prescription drugs paid for if they had a referral from their GP. Contrary to the impression of some Australians that I met, patients can move from one GP to another. Further, this registration has subsequently provided major benefits in terms of monitoring health and health promotion.

Within such a system, individual GPs received their entire income from the NHS and were remunerated through a mixed system that combined a salary with capitation based simply on the number of patients on a doctor's list.

Then, with the 1991 reform, the concept of GP fund-holding was introduced. The purpose of this system was to give incentives to GPs to provide the most cost-effective form of care. Under the system of fund-holding, GPs were given a 'fund' made of two spending categories: the cost of drugs they prescribed to their patients and the cost of certain kinds of specialist and hospital treatment for their patients. If, during a given period, the actual expenditures were less than the budgeted fund, the GP was allowed to spend the surplus on improvements to their practice. Conversely, GPs who exceeded their budgeted fund faced a penalty corresponding to a portion of their deficit.

One criticism of the fund-holding system was that it tended to produce inequality in the standard of care that different patients groups were receiving. More precisely, GPs in poorer regions had patients with greater healthcare needs than those practising in more affluent areas, making it harder for the former to generate a surplus. Another critique of GP fund-holding was its very high administrative costs: GPs found that negotiating with hospitals and specialists for health services was both cumbersome and time-consuming. By 1997 and the change of government, 50% of all GPs had become fund-holders.

In the 1997 White Paper, the Blair Government reformed the GP fund-holding system by creating primary care groups. PCGs were based upon an alternative model known as local commissioning pilots, which had been developed by groups of GPs concerned about the inequalities caused by fund-holding.

Thus, PCGs were groups of practices covering between 50 000 to 250 000 people in designated geographic areas. They were expected to develop through a number of stages until they were able to assume responsibility for commissioning care and for the provision of community health services for their population. In practice, by April 2002, they had all evolved into primary care trusts and local health authorities had been abolished.

The various reforms enacted throughout the 1990s, such as GP fund-holding and more recently the creation of PCGs, did not affect the ways that general practitioners received their personal incomes. Fund-holding budgets were for the purchase of hospital and community services and could not be used to supplement GPs' incomes. Currently, GPs are paid by the NHS as independent, self-employed professionals under a 'cost-plus' principle – the payments they receive cover their expenses in delivering services (the 'cost') and a net income for doing so (the 'plus'). The basic elements of the current payment system include:

- *Capitation fees* are annual fees payable for each patient registered on their list (with three levels of payment depending on the age of the patient). These amount to just over one-half of GPs' gross income from all fees and allowances.
- *Allowances* are the next largest element for the average GP and include a basic practice allowance that covers the basic costs incurred in setting up and maintaining a practice. The level of this allowance can vary in order to encourage practitioners to locate in under-serviced areas.
- *Health promotion payments* comprise payments for running health promotion and chronic disease management programmes.
- *Item of service payments* are paid every time a GP provides certain, usually preventive, services (e.g. contraception).

Overall, this combination of types of payment means that the income of individual GPs will depend on the number of patients on their list, the fees and allowances for which they qualify, the number and level of activities undertaken and the performance achieved.

It has been a considerable success in incentivising computerisation of general practice and health promotion activity. However, the rapid and recent advent of primary care trusts may finally reduce significantly or even destroy the independent contractor status. In interviews, concern was expressed over the failure of the model to properly address the diverse nature of primary care:

> The PCTs are target driven. The model is based upon secondary care. Many of the things that general practice does never appear in the targets. Many GPs are very disillusioned and I foresee major problems.
> (Former practice manager)

There are approximately 230 independent medical/surgical facilities and hospitals in the United Kingdom. In these private settings, doctors are paid fee-for-service either directly by the patient who may be then reimbursed by a private insurance company if they are a policyholder, or by the private hospital/clinic at which the services are provided. Private sector care is specialised and is mainly used for such elective (non-emergency) surgical procedures as hernias, varicose vein surgery and hip replacements. Abortions are the most common procedure (13.2% of the total). In recent years, there has been substantial growth in rather more complex procedures such as coronary bypass grafts and other heart operations.

A major shift has occurred in recent years. Whilst the NHS has always made some use of privately run hospitals, the current Government made a commitment to be pragmatic after the election as to whether private or public hospitals should be used to treat NHS patients. Those patients would be treated free at the point of use of those services, whether public or private. This was to try to bring down the waiting lists and waiting times, particularly for non-urgent medical treatments, and to help achieve the targets set by the Government.

However, early pilots have demonstrated that the required contractual relationships are complex and are reminiscent of the administrative headaches experienced by GP fund-holders under the old system.

The UK public would identify strongly with the Canadian value of healthcare provided free at the point of care. However, many would find the apparent prohibition on private healthcare puzzling, although it is likely that this would find more favour in Scotland than England (take-up rates of private healthcare insurance in Scotland are one-quarter those in London). On the other hand, Canadians would find the waiting times in the UK system unacceptable.

The Australians would also find the UK system unacceptable in terms of its access to care. We shall return to the issue of choice in primary care in the next chapter.

# What the people say

In preparing this book, a number of interviews were conducted in each country with a variety of people from different perspectives, including clinicians, managers and academics. Formal interviews with professionals were supplemented with more informal conversations with patients.[35]

In the UK, the major themes emerging from the interviews were the following:

- access to care
- change
- the role of doctors
- fragmentation.

# Access to care

Access to care measured as waiting list size remains the dominant measure of quality of care in the UK NHS:

> The chief executive knows that they will lose their job if they don't get waiting lists down. Nothing else, including balancing the books, is a sackable offence if they fail, so the outcome is predictable.
>
> (Doctor)

Following a scandal at the Royal Bath Hospital[36] over falsification of waiting list figures:

> Many chief executives will be quaking in their boots this morning. They're under such pressure over waiting lists that they will do anything to make the figures look good. The dividing line between presentation and falsification is very grey indeed.
>
> (NHS manager)

Respondents talked openly of patients receiving letters taking them off waiting lists after 11 months and methods to delay placing patients onto the waiting lists in the first place.

An example of the tensions caused by this pressure was the rush to recruit staff from overseas whose first language was not English, in spite of communication problems being top of patient complaint lists:

> The nurses brought in were having to be given language lessons, first in English then in local dialect.
>
> (Lecturer working with an NHS trust)

Further tension may be caused by the increased use of day surgery to increase efficiency without adequate after-care in the community:

> She was sent home from hospital, whilst still feeling nauseous and quite incapable of looking after herself. She lived alone with no family to help her and no professional support.
>
> (Outraged friend of elderly day-surgery patient)

Patients generally expect to wait for non-life-threatening conditions but a number commented that by the time they were admitted their condition had significantly worsened:

> It wasn't bothering me, but now it's extremely uncomfortable and I still don't know when they'll do it.
>
> (Patient having waited over 12 months)

In general, patients and professionals were sceptical over the validity of waiting list data and the impact of changes:

> The Prime Minister tells that the patients on my list that have been waiting more than 18 months are a figment of my imagination. What a relief, because I thought there were quite a lot of them!
>
> (Orthopaedic surgeon)

At the time of writing, the official waiting list figures have started to reduce. It remains to be seen how far they will have to reduce to convince the sceptical public and professions.

## Change

Nearly everyone approached agreed that change was a major characteristic of the NHS as an organisation. The rate of change in both processes and organisational structures was cited as a problem and the barrier to improvement:

> First we had two PCGs in the town, then they were amalgamated in a single PCG in preparation for trust status. Most of the staff in the PCG whose Chief Executive lost his job were shocked as they felt that he was

the more dynamic character. Many left after amalgamation, and the others lost much of their motivation.

Just 12 months later we became a PCT and the Chief Executive lost her job and a new appointment was brought in from outside, so any remaining continuity and motivation was destroyed.

(PCT staff member)

There's no money for education and training this year because the PCT has not worked out what it's doing yet.

(Training manager)

At the same time, the patient perspective is that little change has been achieved in key problems areas, notably in access to care:

We still can't get to see our GP.

(Patient)

I've been waiting 15 months for my operation and I still haven't got a date for it.

(Patient)

The Prime Minister has complained about cynicism as a barrier to change, but patients point to the disparity between the vision and the reality:

What's the point of being able to book an appointment for a convenient time, when I can't get an appointment inside 12 months?

(Patient)

The Protti report,[37] commissioned by the Information Policy Unit of the Department of Health, has some interesting insights from the perspective of an external (Canadian) academic:

Returning to the UK, it did not take me long to realise that the NHS was once again in the midst of a significant period of transition. It was evident, even to an outsider, that the United Kingdom has a Government which believes that the NHS has to be reorganised and made to be more equitable, accountable and customer-focused. I sensed that it is a Government that is looking for obvious progress in reforming the public sector – spurred on in particular by negative media coverage about the NHS.

In its recent policy document, *Shifting the Balance of Power in the NHS (StBOP)*, the Government expresses its desire to devolve power and decision making down to the front line, to decentralise, to provide patients with choice, to give local staff the resources and the freedoms to innovate, develop and improve local services. This desire pervades the changes I observed and sets the tone for my report – these are fascinating, if somewhat daunting, times for the NHS.

(Protti report, p.4)

I could not help but sense that many parts of the NHS are feeling beleaguered, micro-managed, under-funded and suffering from a surfeit of 'changeitis'. Many feel that they are constantly in response mode – particularly to requests from the Centre, from Task Forces etc. Few would argue with the objectives of the performance management targets – it is more about the number of them and the pace of change. Some would argue that there is an inconsistency between the empowerment rhetoric in *StBOP* and the day-to-day realities of performance management monitoring. In my opinion, there is a pressing need to reduce the number of developments and initiatives. It would be wise to focus down on a number of key initiatives in the next two years to bolster confidence in what is being done by making demonstrable improvements for NHS staff and patients.

(Protti report, p.6)

It is increasingly self-evident that change management and organizational development activities must accompany the introduction of an electronic care record. While such capabilities may often be 'ahead of the organization', it must not be so far ahead of the process that it causes the organization to give up before the journey is over. Therefore, a key requirement of senior leadership is to carefully manage the trade-off between the healthy changes introduced by the electronic care record and the increased risk that its implementation will fail because of those changes.

(Protti report, p.52)

Whilst this report specifically deals with the introduction of electronic health records (EHRs) into the NHS, this innovation is a key part of improving patient care and a microcosm of the whole organisation. Professor Protti's comments cited here relate to change management within the NHS, not just specifically to EHRs.

# The role of doctors

In spite of the increase in multi-professional working, the focus of the NHS is still very much on the doctors. Some are receptive to change:

As a GP, with a proper team of nurses and other healthcare professionals, I could increase my list size from 2000 to 10 000.

(A former GP, no longer in general practice(!))

Some are less so:

GPs should remain the gatekeepers to the rest of the NHS. Nurses are not qualified to spot the problems that we pick up.

(GP)

More interesting are the perceptions of patients, who tended to describe the medical profession as a whole as:

> arrogant and poor communicators
>
> (Patient)

but would generally offer no criticism of their own doctor:

> He's a saint.
>
> (Same patient)

The reduced status of the profession as a whole has provided opportunities for the Government to introduce a range of measures from formal reaccreditation schemes to the use of monitoring software at the heart of the electronic patient system. Consider for example PROFESS:[38]

> PROFESS is an experimental project to determine the technical feasibility of collecting specific information from primary care practice systems, on a voluntary basis, for the purpose of providing a learning support system through an analysis service to subscribing practices. There is no compulsion to use the system, and the data is pseudonomised so that it is not possible to identify patients or clinicians. The primary purpose of the PROFESS system is to provide analysable information, for use by individual practices to reflect on their own practice information when compared, in an anonymised and secure way, with all participating practices. The analysis provision will help GPs to check, for example, data pertaining to their own patients in specific disease groups such as CHD or diabetes. Another use for the system is that it can be used as an adjunct to PRODIGY, although using PRODIGY does not automatically include the use of PROFESS. When used with PRODIGY, the system can provide information about the use of PRODIGY guidance, which could then be used to inform the future development of PRODIGY guidance in line with perceived patterns of use across all participating practices. The project is currently undergoing technical feasibility and in the process of thorough evaluation. A government and professional ethics committee is also being set up to discuss and ensure the safeguarding of data use.
> (Sowerby Centre for Health Informatics at Newcastle website, 2002)

Its detractors have cited it as an example of spy software, albeit officially endorsed spy software.

It represents an extraordinary philosophical position on the nature of healthcare. It measures what the doctor does against a set of rigid protocols derived as the lowest common denominator from the meta-analysis of a range of trials in a variety of environments. It assumes that if the doctor departs from the guideline this is because he is incompetent rather than because he is overruling the computer because of his own expertise. If we don't have confidence in that expertise, why do we pay doctors as professional experts and not as computer operators?

A thought experiment that I use with students goes as follows:

> *A village GP in his fifties has just installed a new computer system in his surgery. He has practised in the same village all his life and his father before him. Most of his patients have parents who were his patients. A patient enters for a consultation and the doctor calls up the patient's electronic health record. A message pops up on the screen providing the GP with advice from a national guideline. He chooses to ignore it. Why?*
>
> Choose from one of the following answers:
>
> 1 He's past it.
> 2 He doesn't trust the technology.
> 3 He knows his patient and decides that he knows what's best for the patient.
> 4 He weighs up the evidence and on balance decides that the guideline is not appropriate in this case.
>
> (Extract from teaching materials, 2002)

The answers paint the doctor in a range of states from incompetent to expert. Many students in the current environment can be readily persuaded that the most likely answers are the first two.

The only rational basis for paying doctors as professionals is that there are cases where they need to weigh local knowledge, knowledge of patient history and environment and interpret the evidence in the light of it. A system like PROFESS is incapable of making the distinction between answers 1 to 4. The scary part is that it seems to suggest that we believe answer 1 is more likely than answer 4.

In spite of this, and in spite of the impact of scandals discussed in Chapter 10, most patients still trust their doctor.

# Fragmentation

A key complaint was of fragmentation of care. The Government is committed to a seamless, paperless, electronic NHS by 2005. This is in stark contrast to the current situation, characterised by the following comments:

> When we've sorted out the hospital's electronic record system then we'll consider the links to primary care.
>
> (Hospital IT manager)

> It can still take six weeks for a discharge summary to arrive from the hospital.
>
> (GP)

> When a patient moves practice we have no alternative but to print out their electronic record and hope the next practice type it into theirs.
>
> (Practice manager)

More serious still are the barriers between health and social care. A study of information support for integrated care within an NHS mental health trust revealed the following organisational structure:[39]

> The in-patient unit was placed within the general hospital, which was a separate trust. It had 29 acute admission beds, with no separate ward for females. There were three consultant psychiatrists. The staff complement was one ward manager, four sister/charge nurses, eight 'E' grade staff nurses and 16 nursing assistants. Internal rotation was in operation, with four members of night staff, two of which were trained nurses. The complement for day staff was five per shift. There was also an assistant nurse who worked nine to five to assist with patient activities. Until recently the advocacy service 'ACE' (advocate, communication and empowerment) ran individual surgeries for patients; also a pre-discharge group ran on a weekly basis, facilitated by the National Association of Mental Health (MIND). Voluntary groups needed accurate information if they were to represent patients regarding their care and this provided an impetus for staff to collate information that might be required by this service.
>
> The in-patient unit suffered many of the general problems faced within the acute psychiatric services throughout the country and these have been highlighted in a recent publication concerning acute services. The unit was open for 24 hours, seven days per week. Nursing documentation was kept on the ward and when the patient was discharged, the documentation was filed within the back of the medical records.
>
> The CIS (Computerised Information System) was networked on the ward, but the only inputting done by nursing staff was the *Health of the Nation* outcome scores (HoNOS) as the ward was taking a lead position in its piloting within the Trust. The ward, as with every other site at the Trust, was unable to access any other computerised system even though they used the same pathology and X-ray services which had no interface for communication to the ward despite being in the same building.
>
> The day hospital was based below the in-patient unit and offered placement for ten places per day. In-patient groups were also held within the day hospital. The day hospital ran electroconvulsive therapy (ECT) sessions twice per week for the whole service and was required to report to a national data collection study at the Department of Health. The staffing was two full-time trained nurses, with a part-time trained member who ran the ECT sessions.
>
> An occupational therapist (OT) attended the day hospital on a session basis in order to facilitate the needs of the in-patient group who attended these sessions. The OT department provided a separate team based at a nearby hospital. The team covered both the acute and elderly services. Two nursing assistants also worked in day care, with time allocated to out-patients (OP). Both day care services and out-patient services were networked to CIS. This service was only open nine to five, Monday to Friday, with the nursing documentation always kept separate from the in-patient nursing records, causing problems if out-of-hours access was required by the services which covered a 24-hour period. The OTs also kept their own case notes at a separate base.

The 11 community psychiatric nurses (CPNs) were based within one building situated approximately one mile away from the acute psychiatric unit. Their main target group was patients with enduring mental illness, but they also responded to referral from the primary care groups. As with the in-patient unit, they worked within the confines of the Care Programme Approach (CPA). The team provided a nine-to-five service, with weekend cover, also nine to five. The CPN department kept all their documentation within their own filing system at their own site.

The psychology department was once again separately organised, based at a different location. The psychology services received referrals from GPs as well as referrals from the other areas within the Trust. The psychology department had its own systems and did not work within the CPA (DoH, 1990a), but had its own records. The psychologists offered a service that covered the hours of nine to five, Monday to Fridays, as in the case of other services within the Trust; documentation was filed and kept on their own site.

To make things even more confusing, the counselling and psychotherapy teams were based within two further sites, one being in the main town itself and the other based ten miles away. The team had one manager who covered both sites but was based at yet another site. The counselling services took clients mainly from the PCGs, but also had expertise in dealing with enduring mental illness and took referrals from secondary services. The service worked within the CPA (DoH, 1990a). The remote clinic was based upstairs with its reception downstairs. Remarkably, the computerised information system was only networked upstairs, so appointments and referrals were entered onto a stand-alone system downstairs by the receptionist. The service was offered on an appointment basis, nine to five, Monday to Friday. Once again, documentation was kept separately and filed on site.

At the time the Trust had only one self-harm liaison nurse, who was based one mile away from the acute unit. The liaison nurse had time allocated to do initial assessment on the medical wards in the general hospital and worked closely with Accident and Emergency (A&E) and the on-call psychiatrist. He did not use CPA or the risk assessments used within other areas of the Trust (DoH, 1990a). He had his own assessment tool and retained his own documentation. The service he provided was from nine to five, Monday to Friday, and there was no access to his documentation outside of these hours as they were kept locked in his office.

The Drug and Alcohol Consortium was based on yet another site, approximately one mile away from the in-patient unit. It took referrals from primary and secondary services. Alcohol referrals were only accepted via the Alcohol Advisory Service, which was based in a different location in the town. Patients were required to self-refer to the Alcohol Advisory Service. Once again, the Drug and Alcohol Consortium did not work within the guidelines of CPA or risk assessment (DoH, 1990a). They also had their own documentation, which remained on site. The service was offered on a nine-to-five basis, Monday to Friday, with no access to documentation or services outside these hours.

The Intensive Home Support Team (IHST) was not networked to the computer system and stood as a joint team of health staff and social services staff. It was based within the social services resource centre at a different location in the town, approximately two miles away from the in-patient unit. The team worked closely with patients to provide either early discharge support from the in-patient unit or to give intensive support in an attempt to prevent admission. Initially the team worked to provide weekend cover on a nine-to-five basis, seven days a week, but the weekend cover was stopped due to service changes. This team worked within the confines of CPA (DoH, 1990a) and also piloted the use of HoNOS to predict psychiatric morbidity (Wing *et al.*, 1996). The service kept separate records for health staff and social staff 'for legal reasons' on advice from the Trust solicitor.

The mental health social services were also based at the same site as the intensive home care team, which lent itself to some sharing of documentation and information. The service comprised of the purchasing team and the provider team with both teams having different team leaders. The purchasing team completed the referrals to the service using a banding system. If the referral met the banding criteria then it was given to the provider team. There is no other route into the service. If the childcare social work team had a referral for social worker input, then the same referral system would be followed. The social services resource centre had close links with housing and education. They had a day care centre that operated on a nine-to-five basis, Monday to Friday. The mental health social services worked within CPA (DoH, 1990a) but were not networked to CIS. They were networked to the social services information database (SID) and their notes were not available out of hours.

Another group of practitioners, approved social workers (ASWs), were based at the resource centre on a rotational basis between nine to five, however the out-of-hours work was covered by the Emergency Duty Team (EDT). Their area covered the out-of-hours provision for separate services from the whole of South Humber.

Police services were also involved in the care of the mentally ill. The police got involved with problems that arose in the community and the in-patient unit was a place of safety following arrest. Joint working with the police and the criminal justice system was an area of neglect, which was highlighted in the NSF (DoH, 1999). Once again, documentation did not follow the patient nor were the police or probation services linked into the CIS.

The Trust had established a CIS network to facilitate communication between its dispersed locations. As discussed earlier, social services had their own SID system. However, the links provided to this system were limited. None of the agencies outside the Trust, for example PCGs, social services, police, forensic and probation services, could access the CIS. The Trust itself could not access the SID and not all services within the Trust could access their own computer network.

---

For reference details, see Goddard *et al.*[39]

Within the same trust, it was found that data collection was prone to excessive duplication (*see* Figure 6.1).

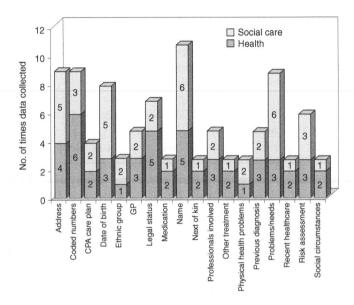

**Figure 6.1** Number of times data collection was duplicated.

Patients were asked their name 11 times during their care and other details such as address nine times. Other more important information such as clinical histories were actually explored much less frequently.

When interviewed, staff working in this environment described their feelings of 'working blind' and attributed this to a range of problems:

- professional tribalism
- concerns over confidentiality
- resistance to change
- lack of basic management data
- lack of basic clinical data
- lack of organisational investment in a unified system.

The Information Commissioner[40] has recently ruled against social care agencies sharing patient information with healthcare colleagues, at least without express consent of the patient. This can only perpetuate the fragmentation of care, which has a major impact on the patient's view of the quality of care:

> The patient came into see me to discuss the results from his hospital visit. He quite reasonably assumed that three weeks after his hospital visit I would have the information and regarded me as a blithering idiot for not knowing what he was talking about!
>
> (GP)

# Conclusions

## Are the policy values carried into practice?

The policy documents emphasise the needs for national standards and cost-effectiveness. There is no doubt that the clinical governance agenda is starting to impact upon the NHS. There is some evidence that access to care is being improved and that waiting times are starting to come down.

At the same time, there is a degree of cynicism about whether the target-driven approach improves overall care or merely improves care in some areas at the expense of others. A clearly communicated view was that the pressure to meet targets was unhelpful and led to practice varying from the unwise to the fraudulent. Another view expressed was that the number of new standards and initiatives was actually a barrier to real improvements in care.

The question of cost-effectiveness is also complex. The NHS is a very cost-effective operation taken as a whole already. The scope for improvements in cost-effectiveness is therefore limited.

The Government's imperative to improve access to care and reduce waiting lists may well reduce cost-effectiveness. It tends to emphasise reduction of waiting lists at almost any cost. The use of Private Finance Initiatives to build and manage new hospitals in an attempt to increase capacity quickly will lead to a long-term reduction in cost-effectiveness of the system.

The lack of integration was highlighted by patients and professionals as a barrier to improving the quality of care. It may also prove a barrier to improving cost-effectiveness as it is impossible to monitor cost and benefits when a cost increase in one sector, e.g. primary care, is more than matched by a saving in another, e.g. secondary care.

# Strengths, weaknesses, opportunities and threats in the UK NHS

The study has revealed the following strengths, weaknesses, opportunities and threats (SWOTs) (*see* Box 6.1).

The fundamental area of weak performance for the UK NHS remains access to care. In the minds of most patients, professionals and politicians, all the rest remains secondary.

The push to get waiting lists down is the one feature which permeates policy and practice. The patients agree that it is the most pressing problem but remain unconvinced of the ability of the NHS to address this fundamental weakness.

At the same time, the quality agenda is being driven by a need to be seen to be responding to the events at Bristol, Alder Hey and other scenes of high-profile scandals.

Ironically, the speed and extent of change is in itself a barrier to improvements.

---

**Box 6.1** SWOTs in the UK NHS

*Strengths*
- Cost-effectiveness
- Patient registration system with GPs
- Health promotion

*Weaknesses*
- Access to care
- Lack of integrated care

*Opportunities*
- Build upon experience to date in EHRs in primary healthcare
- Basic IT infrastructure established through NHSNet
- Inter-professional working

*Threats*
- Cost control within a global economic downturn
- Staff retention and recruitment
- Organisational change
- Litigation as a pressure to defensive behaviour
- Inappropriate targets driving primary care

# CHAPTER 7

# What is the reality in Australia?

## Historical development

The Australian post-war healthcare system differed substantially from that of the UK. Crucially, there was always a significant input from the private sector. The role of the Government was to regulate the market. In 1953, for example, the National Health Act established the fundamental principles of fairness, ensuring for example:

- a common carrier regulation, outlawing discrimination on the grounds of age, sex and health status
- community rating of premiums, to ensure that premiums were set according to communities and not according to an individual's risk. This effectively guaranteed a degree of risk sharing amongst a community. In this case the community was defined as a State.

Just as the UK has reformed the NHS, but never moved fundamentally away from a system dominated by the public sector, so Australia increased or decreased the extent of market involvement. However, there was no move away fundamentally from a regulated market system until a 1974 reform plan that introduced a universal public insurance plan.

The private insurance companies and the Australian Medical Association opposed this change and the universal public plan, much more akin to the Canadian or UK model, lasted less than a year. Its lasting legacy was, however, an increased level of public financing.

The next attempt to introduce a universal healthcare programme was in 1984. This Medicare plan reduced the role of private insurance although, as in the UK, the private insurers continued to offer hospital in-patient insurance to cover services duplicated in Medicare.

However, in 1986 the Government removed subsidies to the private insurers, leading to a rise in premiums in the late 1980s, with a consequent decrease in the uptake of insurance. In 1974 before the first universal plan, the levels of insurance uptake were 80%, and by the mid 1990s had fallen to under one-third.[41] The minority report of the Australian Labour Party[42] into the Private Health Insurance Incentives Bill 1998 and related bills cites a figure of 15% by 1998.

# The current situation

The Australian Doctors' Reform Society provides the following summary of the state of Australian health:[43–46]

> Australians enjoy a high overall level of population health status on almost every criterion. Most measures of death and illness show Australia ranks in the middle range of developed countries. For example, age-standardised death rates take into account the different age distributions across countries. Comparing the number of deaths per 100 000 people provides a comparison of a nation's overall health status. In 1992, Australia had the fifth lowest rate among 19 comparable developed countries, ahead of the UK and bettered only by Japan, Hong Kong, Sweden and Canada. Australia's death rate was 16% lower than the rates for the USA and New Zealand, which ranked 15th and 16th respectively.
>
> Life expectancy in Australia in 1996 was 78.2 years, one year greater than the OECD [Organisation for Economic Cooperation and Development] median and 2.1 years more than the USA – while infant mortality was equal to the OECD median of 5.8 per 1000 live births, roughly comparable with Canada and better than the UK.
>
> In 1995, a comparison of eight developed countries ranked Australia second only to Japan in achieving the lowest potential years of life lost for all causes except suicide for people under the age of 70.
>
> (Medicare Fact Sheet 6, *How Australia's Health*
> *Service Compares Internationally*)

Like Canada, Australia has a federal system of government and responsibility for healthcare is shared between the national (or Commonwealth) Government and sub-national governments (six States and two Territories). In Australia, however, the Commonwealth Government has a stronger role in healthcare than in Canada. While provincial governments in Canada have far greater fiscal leverage in healthcare than does the Federal Government, States and Territories in Australia are largely dependent on the Commonwealth Government for healthcare funding. As in Canada, local governments (municipalities) in Australia play a relatively small role in healthcare.

The Federal (Commonwealth) Government is responsible for public policy making at national level in the fields of public health, research and national health information management. The Commonwealth Government operates the national, publicly funded healthcare insurance plan in Australia, and regulates the private healthcare insurance industry. It also finances and regulates residential aged care (nursing homes) and, jointly with States and Territories, it funds and administers some community-based care and home care. Commonwealth funding for healthcare is derived from general taxation plus a dedicated healthcare levy of 1.5% on taxable income.

The State and Territory governments have primary responsibility for the management and delivery of publicly insured health services within their jurisdiction. As such, they deliver public acute and psychiatric hospital services and a wide range of community and public health services, including school health, dental care, maternal and child health. State and Territory governments are also responsible for the regulation of healthcare providers as well as for the licensing and approval of private hospitals. Healthcare funding by States and Territories is derived mostly from grants from the Commonwealth Government as well as from general taxation and user charges.

Health promotion and disease prevention programmes (such as immunisation) and environmental health services (such as sanitation and hygiene) are organised at a local level.

The national, publicly funded healthcare insurance plan in Australia, known as Medicare, is a compulsory scheme that provides universal coverage for all. Public healthcare insurance is broader in Australia than in Canada as it covers physicians, hospitals, prescription drugs and some community-based care and home care. However, user charges and extra billing are frequently required for publicly insured health services.

Thus, whilst Medicare covers a GP consultation, Australians may choose one of three options. They may visit a block-billing GP who will bill the Government under Medicare, and thus the consultation is 'free' to the patient. They may visit a GP who charges them but only at a rate that they can reclaim at a later date. Thus they have to put money out, but will get it back. Their third choice is to visit a GP who charges more than the Government will reimburse, in which case they can reclaim only a portion of the cost.

This situation, which appears quite foreign to patients in the UK or Canada, arises from the structure of Australian Medicare, which is made up of three parts:

1 The *Medical Benefits Scheme* (MBS) ensures access to physician services (outside of hospitals). The MBS lists a wide range of physician services and stipulates the fee applicable to each item (the 'scheduled fee'). The MBS reimburses only 85% of the doctor's scheduled fee. In other words, Australian physicians may extra bill. When doctors bill Medicare directly ('bulk bill'), they accept the 85% level as full payment and the patient pays nothing. When doctors charge more than the scheduled fee, the patient must pay the difference between the Medicare benefit and the scheduled fee and then claim reimbursement from Medicare or alternatively obtain from Medicare a cheque made out to the physician. However, a safety net provision applies to MBS: once patients have paid a certain fee in physician fees in a given year they are exempt from further charges. Private insurance is not allowed to provide coverage for physician services that are publicly insured or for the gap between Medicare and the fee charged by the doctor. Some categories of patients (mostly social security recipients and veterans) are not required to pay any extra billing.

2 The *Australian Health Care Arrangements* (AHCAs) provide the basis for funding by the Commonwealth Government to the States and Territories for hospital services. Funding by the Commonwealth Government takes the form of annual block grants whose amounts are negotiated in five-year agreements with the States and Territories, who in return agree not to allow user charges for public hospital services. The extent of public coverage for hospital care depends on whether a patient elects to be a public patient or a private patient. Full coverage for hospital care is provided to public patients in State- and Territory-owned hospitals or in private, non-profit hospitals. Public patients are also entitled to free hospital care in for-profit hospitals which have made arrangements with governments to care for public patients. However, when an individual chooses

to be a private patient in a public hospital (in which case they have the ability to choose their own doctor) or goes to a private hospital, the Commonwealth Government pays only 75% of the scheduled hospital-based physician fee. All other costs are the responsibility of the patient. The safety net that applies to physician services under the MBS and which limits the amount paid by the patient in a one-year period does not apply to Medicare benefits for hospital services. Private healthcare insurance is allowed to cover the difference between 75% of the scheduled fee and the actual fee charged. Private insurers can also provide additional benefits for hospital accommodation and other hospital charges.

3 The *Pharmaceutical Benefits Scheme* (PBS), which is based on a national drug formulary, provides free access to drugs prescribed outside of hospital, subject to annual thresholds. Under the PBS, eligible people fall into two categories: general patients and concessional patients. General patients are required to pay a charge per prescription up to an annual threshold; beyond that limit, they are required to pay only a much smaller small charge per prescription. Concessional card-holders pay the smaller charge per prescription until they reach a much lower threshold, after which their drugs are fully paid by the Commonwealth. If the prescription involves a more costly but equivalent brand, the subsidy may be limited to the lower cost brand (this is called the minimum pricing policy). Individuals must pay for drugs not listed on the national formulary in full and, also in full, for drugs that are priced below the co-payment amount. It is estimated that about 75% of all prescriptions issued in Australia are subsidised under the PBS.

As in Canada, some services are not covered under Australian Medicare, such as cosmetic surgery, and services provided under workers' compensation insurance and private insurance can cover allied health/paramedical services (such as physiotherapists' and podiatrists' services) as well as some aids and devices. However, in contrast to Canada, private healthcare insurance in Australia both complements and competes with Medicare since private insurers may cover the same benefits as under the public plan. Australians can supplement their Medicare benefits through private healthcare insurance, but they cannot opt out of the publicly funded system since they continue to pay their taxes.

Defenders of the private healthcare system in Australia point to the safeguards:[47]

> Health insurance in Australia is fully community rated, which I think reflects its social role as far as governments are concerned. By 'fully community rated' I mean that there is no premium discrimination against people by virtue of age, sex, state of health or potential health risk. The only restriction is a 12-month waiting period after joining for pre-existing ailments. At the end of 12 months, benefits are fully payable for pre-existing conditions as well as for conditions that occur after joining. I think you can see from that that there is a very strong social component of the private sector in Australia, and it does link in quite well with the public sector.
>
> (Russell Schneider, Chief Executive Officer,
> Australian Health Insurance Association)

The Commonwealth Government is responsible for regulating private healthcare insurance and it retains the principle that premiums be community rated. This means that private insurers must establish a common premium structure for all enrolees, regardless of their health status. In other words, they cannot charge higher rates for high-risk individuals such as the aged or the chronically ill. Community rating ensures that private insurance is available to a wide range of people in the community. This in turn necessitates a system of re-insurance, designed to ensure that insurers with high proportions of aged and chronically ill customers do not suffer competitive disadvantage. The Commonwealth Government has also introduced a number of tax-based measures to encourage people to purchase private healthcare insurance in order to counteract a long-term trend of decreasing take-up of private insurance. Overall, there are about 40 private healthcare insurance funds registered in Australia.

As in Canada, some 70% of healthcare spending is financed by the public sector (46% by the Commonwealth Government and 24% by State and Territory governments) and 30% by the private sector. This is a significantly higher percentage than in the UK, where the percentage of private expenditure is nearer to 20% of the whole. We shall return to this apparent paradox that the Canadian system has as high a percentage of private expenditure as the Australian system in the next chapter.

The greater role of the Commonwealth Government in Australia when compared with the Federal Government in Canada is reflected in the proportion of finances coming from the national centre. The Commonwealth Government in Australia is the primary public insurer of prescription drugs and physician services. It also funds some 50% of hospital expenditures.

Medicare is financed largely by general taxation revenue, some of which is raised by an income-related Medicare levy at the national level. This Medicare levy is paid by individuals at a basic rate of 1.5% of taxable income above certain income thresholds. Individuals who do not pay any income tax do not pay the Medicare levy (but they are entitled to full coverage under Australian Medicare). Taxpayers with high incomes who do not have private healthcare insurance pay an additional 1% of taxable income as part of the levy. The Medicare levy accounts for approximately 27% of Commonwealth funding for Medicare and for about 8% of total healthcare spending in Australia.

As in Canada, and in the primary care sector of the UK, the majority of doctors are self-employed. Most primary care provided by GPs in private practice is reimbursed on a fee-for-service basis. A small proportion of physicians are salaried employees of Commonwealth, State/Territory or local governments. General practitioners in primary care act as gatekeepers, with access to specialist medical services being available only on their referral.

Hospital care is provided by a mix of public and private institutions. In 1999–2000 there were 748 public hospitals nationally, including 24 psychiatric hospitals, compared with 756 in 1995–96. There was an average of 52 947 beds in public hospitals during 1999–2000, representing 68% of all beds in the hospital sector (public and private hospitals combined). Public hospital beds have declined from 3.3 beds per 1000 population in 1995–96 to 2.8 beds in 1999–2000.

The number of patient separations (discharges, deaths and transfers) from public hospitals during 1999–2000 was 3.9 million, compared with 3.6 million in 1995–96. Same-day separations accounted for 46% of total separations in 1999–2000 compared with 40% in 1995–96. Total days of hospitalisation for public health patients during 1999–2000 amounted to 16.2 million, a decrease of 2% since 1995–96. The average length of hospital stay per patient in 1999–2000 was 4.2 days. For 1995–96 the corresponding figure was 4.6, reflecting the lower numbers of same-day patients compared with 1999–2000. If same-day patients are excluded, the 1999–2000 average length of stay was 6.9 days, compared with 7.0 days in 1995–96.

An average of 175 291 staff (full-time equivalent) were employed at public hospitals in 1999–2000, of whom 45% were nursing staff and 10% were salaried medical officers. Revenue amounted to $1223m. Most of this revenue (59%) was from patients' fees and charges. Recurrent expenditure amounted to $14 350m, of which 62% was for salaries and wages. The difference between revenue and expenditure is made up by payments from State/Territory consolidated revenue and specific payments from the Commonwealth for public hospitals, in roughly equal proportions.

There were 509 private hospitals in operation in 1999–2000, comprising 278 acute hospitals, 24 psychiatric hospitals and 207 free-standing day hospital facilities. The number of acute and psychiatric hospitals has continued to decline since 1995–96 when 323 of these hospitals were in operation. In contrast, day hospital facilities have shown strong growth for several years, with only 140 in operation in 1995–96.

The average number of beds available at private acute and psychiatric hospitals for admitted patients increased by 4% to 23 665 between 1995–96 and 1999–2000. Although there was a slight decrease in the average number of beds from 1998–99, the trend towards larger hospitals continues. There were 1.2 private hospital beds available per 1000 population in 1999–2000. The average number of beds or chairs at free-standing day hospital facilities (used mainly for short post-operative recovery periods) increased over the same five-year period by 55% to 1581. This large increase reflects the substantial growth in the numbers of free-standing day hospitals in recent years.

Private hospital separations in 1999–2000 totalled 2.1 million, of which 84% were from private acute and psychiatric hospitals and 16% from free-standing day hospital facilities. Same-day separations accounted for 56% of all private hospital separations (compared with 46% of public hospital separations). This higher proportion of same-day separations contributed to the lower average length of stay in private hospitals (3.2 days) compared to public hospitals (4.2 days).

Public hospitals remain the major providers of care. Public hospitals include hospitals established by State/Territory governments and hospitals established by religious or charitable bodies but now directly funded by government (private non-profit hospitals). Specialists in public hospitals are either salaried or paid on a per-session basis. Salaried specialist doctors in public hospitals can treat some patients in these hospitals as private patients, charging fees to those patients and usually contributing some of their fee income to the hospital.

There are a small number of private for-profit hospitals built and managed by private firms providing public hospital services under arrangements with State/Territory governments. However, most acute care beds and emergency out-patient clinics are in public hospitals.

Private hospitals tend to provide less complex non-emergency care, such as simple elective surgery. However, some private hospitals are increasingly providing complex, high-technology services. Like public hospitals, some private facilities provide same-day surgery and other non-in-patient operating room procedures. Public and private hospitals are not perfect substitutes for each other, however, as accident and emergency facilities, as well as technologically complex and highly specialised services, remain concentrated in the public sector.

A significant proportion of other healthcare providers are self-employed. In addition, there are many independent pathology and diagnostic imaging services operated by doctors.

Australia shares many similarities with Canada: both countries have the same political system of government, they have similar geography and they enjoy similar health outcomes. They also share similar healthcare problems, with significant indigenous populations with particular healthcare needs and large rural areas with sparse populations. The public share of total healthcare spending is the same in Canada as in Australia (around 70%). However, Australia manages to spend much less on healthcare as a percentage of GDP (8.5%) than does Canada (9.5%). Australian Medicare is a single national programme, whereas Canadian Medicare is an amalgam of separate provincial and territorial healthcare insurance plans. In Australia, the national Government plays a stronger role in healthcare than does its Canadian counterpart and it is more able to take unilateral action when reforms are undertaken.

In Australia, the Commonwealth Government operates a national Pharmacare programme, the PBS. It is the view of the Commonwealth Government that the PBS has succeeded in containing the cost of prescription drugs for a number of reasons. First, since 1993, the PBS does not list a drug on its formulary unless it receives a positive assessment with respect to safety, quality, effectiveness and cost-effectiveness. This is analogous to the role of NICE in the UK system, in refusing to allow the prescription of drugs which may be shown to be safe but where cost-effectiveness is not proven.

Second, higher user charges are required for brand-name drugs when generic copies are available. Third, a 'reference pricing' mechanism ensures that the Government subsidises only up to the price of a lower-priced drug that is therapeutically interchangeable with, or equivalent to, the prescribed drug. Overall, the PBS subsidises about 75% of all prescriptions in Australia, and the average subsidy is 57% of the prescription cost.

Ambulance services in Australia are privately operated and require Australians to carry separate ambulance insurance cover.

In a fundamental difference from the UK and Canada, physicians in Australia may extra bill. Therefore, they are not wholly dependent on the Government for remuneration. They can bill patients at rates of their own choosing above the scheduled fee. One implication of this is that Australian GPs have accepted a considerably lower level of public remuneration than is the case in Canada.

The current Government has sought to reverse the traditional decline in the uptake of private health insurance. They have clearly indicated that they believe that a healthy private sector has beneficial effects:[48]

> Yet, this additional funding for public hospitals will only be a stopgap if nothing further is done to support the viability of the private health sector and to address the reasons for the drop-out from private health insurance. The truth is we know the principal reason why people are dropping out of private health insurance and that is the problem of

cost. In fact, to fail to do anything to address these crucial issues would be unreasonable and simply short-sighted. To do nothing could well spell the end of the private sector and only lead to increasing and intolerable strains on the public sector. That's why, Mr Speaker, it would be a serious mistake if this legislation were blocked or delayed.

It would also be a serious miscalculation to assume that the same amount of money would be better spent elsewhere in the public hospital system. Those views are flawed because they haven't taken into account that, in the latest healthcare agreements recently signed with the States, every time health insurance levels drop one per cent, the Commonwealth has to pay the States $83 million more.

Given that those who argue against this rebate are not proposing doing anything and will simply put private health on the back-burner, we can safely assume that the drop-out rate from private health insurance will follow the long-term trend line of two per cent a year.

So by July 2001, if nothing were done, the Government would have to find exactly $500 million extra to the States. In other words, in three years' time, we will be where we are now – and even worse, will have failed to address one of the root causes of the problem. This 30 per cent cut in private health insurance will make a genuine and lasting difference and will preserve the integrity of our healthcare system, of Medicare and of the public hospitals.

> (The Hon. Dr Michael Wooldridge,
> Minister for Health and Aged Care)

As a consequence, it has provided strong incentives for Australian residents to acquire private healthcare insurance. More specifically, it offers holders of private healthcare insurance a subsidy of 30% of the cost of that insurance. This rebate for private insurance premiums is available to all, regardless of income, as a 30% refundable tax credit. The objective of the Commonwealth Government is to have about one-third of the population participate in private insurance schemes.

It was suggested to me that these incentives actually make it cheaper for some people to have private insurance than not to.

Since July 2000, the 30% rebate legislation stipulates that the private insurance company must offer policies with no gaps between the medical scheduled fee and the fee charged by doctors. This provision, called the 'no gap/known gap', is intended to reduce the gaps and to make the extra charges known to patients. Prior to that reform, private insurance covered only scheduled medical fees and actual fee charges could be much higher: two patients could be given exactly the same treatment for which the private patient received a large bill not reimbursed by private insurance, while the publicly insured patient never saw a bill.

Ironically, this reform introduced by the Government to increase the uptake of private insurance was attacked by some of my respondents as fundamentally reducing the choice of patients to pay more to receive allegedly better care.

A 'Lifetime Health Cover' was also introduced in July 2000. Under this system, individuals aged 30 years or less who purchase private healthcare insurance pay lower premiums throughout their life compared with someone who joins later in life. Over the age of 30, a 2% increase in premiums over the base rate is tacked on for every year a person delays in joining. This initiative is expected to reduce premium rates by encouraging more younger and healthier people to take out private insurance and by discouraging people from joining prior to treatment and leaving following the treatment.

A number of authors have suggested a very large public subsidy for private healthcare insurance may not be an effective use of public funds.[41] They suggest that directing an equivalent expenditure toward public treatment in public hospitals would be more effective.

A representative from the Australian Medical Association, in evidence to the Canadian Romanow Commission, suggested that private insurance for hospital services in Australia has resulted in rationing in the public system (in the form of longer waiting times) and in queue jumping:[47]

> There is more rationing in the public sector. People do not get access. It is very common to meet someone who has waited five years to get a hip replacement or even longer for a knee replacement. There is a lot of rationing in the public sector. We call private health insurance 'queue-jumping insurance'. Basically, it buys a place further up the queue. That is the reality and that is why people like it. They can jump queues if they have the money to do so.

More public funding was provided to deal with longer waiting lists. According to the CEO of the Australian Health Insurance Association, this did not solve the problem:

> Waiting lists at public hospitals are a political problem that varies from time to time. Governments have tried to solve the problem by putting more financial resources into the public sector, but the tendency seems to be the same as it is anywhere else in the world. More money does not reduce waiting lists. All it does is allow those people who were not on the waiting list before to get put on to it.

Those in Canada and the UK who believe in the twin-track private–public system will find comfort in the following view:[47]

> Our experience is every time the State Government announces a programme to deal with waiting times, the waiting times get longer. Because we have this ability within the system to switch from the public to the private and back again, each time the Government says it will spend more money to reduce the waiting lists, expectations of service in the public sector increase and people then rejoin the public sector lists. In reality, programmes to reduce waiting times do not work; they only relocate the business in the public sector.
>
> One of the difficulties is that all non-hospital medical treatment is funded by a single source, which is the Government, and possibly a patient care payment. Health insurance does not apply to non-hospital medical treatment. That leads to some perverse incentives within the system because from both the doctor's point of view and the patient's point of view, the level of rebate for a particular service will be greater if that service is performed in an in-hospital setting, than if that same

service were performed outside the hospital. That could probably be a criticism of our system.

It also makes it difficult for insurers to exercise effective cost containment by the support of primary care interventions, or primary care treatment, for their populations. Consequently, there is a defect in the system. This is a very politically controversial statement, but we would achieve a better healthcare system if we were able to redirect the energies of the private sector and the public sector into primary care interventions, rather than funding high-cost, high-tech hospitalisation, which is where insurers are confined at the moment.

(A representative from the Australian Medical Association,<br>in evidence to the Canadian Romanow Commission)

One of the principal arguments against the increasing role of the private sector is the higher costs associated with private provision compared with the public sector. Much of the data on which this is based are drawn from the United States. Every OECD nation's health spending has risen since 1970. However, where the public sector dominates the market, such as in Australia and the UK, cost rises have been slower and more controlled. In Australia the cost of healthcare has been relatively stable for the past ten years.

Australia's proportion of GDP on health went from 5.2% to 8.4% between 1970 and 1995 while in the USA it rose from 7.4% to 14.5% over the same period. The USA rate has only plateaued in the 1990s, mainly as a result of bureaucratic 'managed care' restrictions on the supply of medical services, something Australia has so far avoided.

Australia's total spending on healthcare, as a proportion of GDP and in the proportion coming from the public sector, ranks in the middle of the developed countries for which data are available.

Note that the USA, with only 46.7% of its healthcare expenditure in the public sector, spends 67% more than Australia as a proportion of GDP and 2.3 times as much per capita.[44] Yet despite this additional spending, the USA reports a worse population health status and has 40 million people without any form of health insurance. Most of its highest spending simply goes on higher costs.

A significant difference between the USA and Australia is the extent of health coverage. All three countries considered in this book espouse the principle of universal health insurance cover, ensuring that all people have access to medical band hospital care when they need it.

Countries which rely more on private funding of healthcare, such as the USA, emphasise the right of individuals to choose how their healthcare needs are met. But in reality, choice is determined by personal wealth. Around 40 million Americans or 16% of the population remain uninsured. For them, the choice may be limited to using dwindling public services, bankruptcy or going without needed care.

The Australian Doctors' Reform Society argues that the Australian system offers greater choice than systems such as the UK NHS, whilst retaining the basic principles of fairness and universality:[43]

The UK's National Health Service provides universal healthcare cover, but offers only limited choice. In international terms, this system is efficient in terms of health outcomes, and fair, because nearly all health-care is paid for by progressive taxation.

(Medicare Fact Sheet 6, *How Australia's Health Service Compares Internationally*)

A Canadian study[41] estimates that the cost of the current Government's incentives for private healthcare insurance is approximately $2.2 billion Au. Savings to the public hospital system are estimated to amount to $0.8 billion Au, leaving a cost of $1.4 billion with little evidence of improved waiting times.

To an outsider, the price of increased choice looks unreasonably high. To gain further insight, we shall consider first the quality issues that are concerning national policy, then the issues raised by the people in the system.

# What the people say

Interviews in Australia involved people from three states and included managers, clinicians and academics. As in the UK, these were complemented by more informal discussions with patients.

The major themes emerging from these discussions were:

- choice
- the role of GPs
- the problems of rural populations.

# Choice

One key theme of Australian respondents was the element of choice within their system:

> That's been one of the strengths of the Australian system up till now: that there is much much more choice here than there is in the UK.
>
> (Hospital manager)

Australian patients do not have a registered GP, and many regarded such a system as an infringement of their personal choice. Instead they generally visit a variety of GPs according to their specific need:

> They will have a really good GP who they really want and that's their primary GP who is generally far too busy, who doesn't necessarily run his practice very economically and who they have to wait for, and so that's the person that they will go to when they are in real trouble.
>
> Then they go to the clinic or out-clinic for a quick script and then maybe they have a separate GP for when they need to go and talk about their venereal disease or a mental health problem.
>
> It's not uncommon to have that range of GPs and of course none of them talk to each other – none of them share records.
>
> (Hospital manager)

This appears as anarchy to a UK-centric academic who is currently struggling to convince the UK NHS to become more joined up. When I suggested to one interviewee that the same result could be achieved within a UK group practice with the benefits of a single primary healthcare record at no charge to the patient, they responded that as a patient they liked the convenience of:

> being able to pop out of the office at lunchtime in the city to visit a doctor, miles from the regular doctor at home in the suburbs.
>
> (Hospital administrator)

In an informal conversation with a patient, they noted that:

> In general, I can choose when I have a hospital procedure and which doctor I have.
>
> (Patient)

However, patient choice may not be as great as it appears. The problem of rural populations is discussed below. Even in urban areas, the doctors may be acting in directions that are restricting patient choice, and we explore this further in the next section.

## The role of GPs

Australian doctors, especially general practitioners, are fiercely independent. On a visit to interview the CEO of a Division of Primary Care,[49] I met an elderly man whose age I estimated to be around 75. He told me:

> I was a doctor in the bush, and my father before me. When I was growing up, we used to toss a coin to see who would do the surgery and who would do the anaesthetic!

He was still practising medicine. Most Australian GPs have practices in suburban areas, but this kind of pioneering spirit never seemed too far away in the interviews I carried out.

Australian GPs were convinced that they were more independent than their UK counterparts:

> We're self-employed business people, not like UK GPs who are NHS employees.
>
> (GP)

The Divisions were set up to support general practice. The stated objectives of the Division I visited were:

1 Increase the amount and level of GP involvement in the activities of the Division.
2 Meet GP continuing medical education (CME) and training needs.
3 Encourage and facilitate linkages between GPs and their communities.
4 Plan and implement divisional activities to address identified health population needs.

5 Promote sustainable health promotion and preventative strategies to patients and the community through local GPs.
6 Maintain an organisational structure that is responsive to change.
7 Facilitate communication between GPs, the Division and other agencies.
8 Promote the health and wellbeing of general practitioners to general practitioners.
9 Provide advocacy on behalf of general practitioners to a variety of bodies and organisations.
10 Undertake the collection, collation and evaluation of data related to identified population health needs.

The CEO described the history and purpose of the Divisions thus:

> In 1993–94 the Government divided Australia up geographically into 120 areas which they called Divisions. The GPs in practice within each geographical area belong to that Division and the reasons for it are many and varied, but there was some political reason about if they wanted a stranglehold of the AMA [Australian Medical Association] and to introduce a new force at the workplace level, which is what Divisions are.
>
> We are not a political organisation, we are not an industrial organisation, we are a professional organisation, in a sense that the College [the RACGP] sets standards and all of that. Our job is to train and support GPs and make them more efficient, make them in theory the big, underlying reason for Divisions to better integrate GPs into the local community. That's the bottom underlying thing, and to work towards more cohesive population health level activities; so instead of having to speak directly, when it doesn't want to, to 20 000 GPs or whatever, the Government talks to the GPs via 120 Divisions and the Divisions are directly funded from what is called the GP Strategy in Canberra, which is about $350m a year, of which Divisions are about $90m, and then there's things on top of that.
>
> The main strategy was to introduce some sort of cohesiveness at a physically workable level, and as you said when I showed you the map of Australia, each Division. I might contradict myself because some of the west Australian Divisions are bigger than Europe. And there might be 120 GPs in that whole Division. Then you've got, say, Brisbane North Division, which is just one other group in the division and it has 600 GPs in a single Division so you've got one that's bigger than Europe with 80 GPs and you've got one that's smaller than London with 600 GPs.
>
> It's taken a number of years for Divisions to establish themselves and gain credibility, but the GPs see that what we do is provide education and training; we go in and assist them in the practice; run cold time checks on their fridges to make sure they are at the right temperature; we go in there and assist them to download information from Canberra about under-immunised children; we assist the practice managers to start recall and reminder systems. We do very practical things. They don't see us in that role now, they know that we are not an arm of the Government. We are funded by the Government but GPs in Australia

are very touchy, very sensitive about their autonomy, and the one thing
that Divisions are is just aggregations of GPs.

(CEO, Division of General Practice)

However, in spite of their protestations over independence and their sensitivity
over their autonomy, a major trend in Australian general practice has been for GPs
to sell their practice to commercial corporations:

> All GPs here are private practitioners. That's not true at another level
> because in reality they are mainly paid out of the public bursary, and
> increasingly there are corporate GPs and corporate medicine has become
> very big here. About 30–40% of all GPs in Western Australia for instance
> are now essentially owned by the corporation; and that is going to be a
> very interesting change because the average GP is valued at about $5m
> per year in terms of their capacity, and the business part of the corpora-
> tion policy in Australia now is to sign up as many GPs as possible and
> then ultimately to get them using the corporate radiology, pathology
> and other practitioners, so that in fact you keep all the money that is
> primarily paid out of the public purse within a particular corporation.
>
> (Hospital quality manager)

Dr Tim Woodruff reported the following in an editorial of the journal of the
Doctors' Reform Society:[50]

> Corporatised medical centres have been around for some decades now
> and despite major concerns when they were introduced, have not been
> expanding in their market share until recently. However, there has been
> a recent change in this pattern with figures suggesting that over 30% of
> GPs in Perth, Melbourne and Sydney are now in some type of cor-
> porate centre. For the purposes of this discussion I would like to
> take the example of the buy-out model. This is the most worrying of
> the models as it appears to have the most potential for harm to patient
> care, costs to patients and costs to taxpayers.
>
> In this model a GP is offered an upfront fee by the corporation which
> may be called goodwill and which is a percentage of the gross earnings.
> The GP is then paid either a salary or a percentage of generated revenue
> and the owners take the rest. The medical centre has GPs, specialists,
> pathology, radiology, pharmacy, physiotherapy and other allied health
> services on site.
>
> Such a medical centre has advantages for the patients and for the
> doctor. For the patients the advantages include:
>
> - co-location of services
> - 24-hour cover
> - comprehensive cover.
>
> For the doctor, advantages include:
>
> - reduced or absent administration fees

- cover for after hours/holidays/other leave
- access to support staff, e.g. nurse etc.
- increased accessibility/communication to specialists, allied health
- upfront goodwill.

However, this model raises several interlinked concerns. There is excellent evidence now available to indicate that patients treated in a fee-for-service environment receive more procedures than those treated in the public system. One could argue that this is due to either under-servicing of public patients, over-servicing of private patients, or a mixture of both. The latter is by far the most likely.

This issue was explored further with the interviewee above:

> Once you start referring through the same people in the whole business – essentially you know, you are on a wonderful little roundabout, whereby you know, you refer to a particular radiologist and that person refers to somebody else and the pathologist gets involved and you know you can see how the money just …
>
> (Hospital quality manager)

**AG:** Are there any ethical concerns raised about this?

> Well, of course there are. All of the companies say that they don't do this. All the GPs say they don't do this. The problem is what happens when you get a significant monopoly. OK, you may not be doing it, but it just so happens that you know your patient is most conveniently going to a pathology practice down the road that happens to be from the same business ultimately.
>
> (Hospital quality manager)

**AG:** There must be large areas in Australia where this happens. This was the problem in the internal market in the UK. As far as the GP being able to choose which hospital he is going to refer you to …

> Yes, that's right and that's obviously going to happen. The corporations at the moment are trying to tie up as many GPs as possible and they are being really quite aggressive at the moment, and they are offering GPs quite generous packages – more than the GPs could earn being a single-handed GP. They are offering them quite good conditions and you know a lot of GPs are perfectly naturally signing up. It's very popular because they make so much money, and a significant number have now been sold and it is my understanding that they offered good rates. The problem is then what happens to the next generation of radiologists who have only the corporate practices to work in. So it is going to be interesting.
>
> (Hospital quality manager)

In an informal conversation with a radiologist, she indicated some of the problems from the supply side:

> I worked for a small radiology clinic that was taken over by a conglo-merate. They vastly underestimated the demand and as a result we were swamped, and the quality of the work which had been very high suffered.
>
> (Radiologist)

A number of interviewees commented upon public resistance to any attempt by the Government to establish a centralised records system based upon a unique identifier:

> A few years ago we tried to introduce a system called the Australia Card. It was a disaster.
>
> (GP)

During early 1985, the Federal Government embarked upon a campaign to address the problems of widespread tax evasion and tax avoidance. The draft White Paper on Tax Reform which was released in the lead-up to the ill-fated Tax Summit in July 1985 mentioned, in a few words, the possibility of a 'national identification system'.

The scheme was developed during the period May 1985 to October 1986. The Senate forced the matter to be referred to a Joint Select Committee of Federal Parliament which considered it in the period December 1985 to March 1986. Public comment to that Committee was severely constrained by the failure of the Government to publish its significantly changed and further developed proposals until after the closing data for public submissions. Despite this, a majority of the Committee, comprising members from all parties, concluded that the scheme should not be proceeded with. The Government ignored that conclusion.

During the early months of the campaign, public opinion polls showed significant support for the scheme. The questions were of the form 'The Government proposes to introduce an Australia Card to address the problems of tax evasion, welfare fraud and immigration. Are you in favour of such a card?'. The fact that some 25–30% of the samples said no to this heavily biased question may reflect considerable cynicism in the community about Government power.

By the beginning of 1986 the Australian Democrats, through their incoming leader Janine Haines, were committed to oppose the scheme. By late 1986 there was greater awareness in the community concerning the scheme and a moderate level of concern. This made it possible for the Shadow Health Minister, James Porter, to convince the Liberal and National Parties (some of whose members had originally been attracted by the scheme) to oppose it. This they did, in the Senate in November–December 1986, with great vigour. The combined strength of the Democrats, Liberals and Nationals defeated the bill.

The scheme comprises a number of inter-dependent elements:

- a central register containing data about each member of the entire population. This would be maintained by the Health Insurance Commission (HIC), which hitherto has been responsible for the Medicare and Medibank private health insurance schemes

- a unique identifying code for each member of the population, which would be assigned by the HIC
- an obligatory, multi-purpose identification card for each member of the population, which would be issued by the HIC
- obligations on individuals to produce the card when undertaking a wide variety of dealings with a wide variety of both government agencies and private sector organisations, including all employers and financial institutions, but also hospitals, real estate agents, produce agents etc.
- obligations on organisations to demand the card, record the code, apply sanctions to people who fail to produce it and report information using the code
- use of the code by a wide variety of organisations. Despite promises to the contrary, it does not appear that private sector record keepers are precluded from using the code as an internal identifier
- use of the register or information from the register by the participating agencies:
  - the Tax Office
  - the Department of Social Security
  - the HIC in respect of both Medicare and the national identification scheme and other agencies:
  - the Immigration Department in specific circumstances
  - the Federal Police in specific circumstances
- use of reports containing the code by the Tax Office
- cross-notification of changes to identifying data, particularly address, between the HIC and the participating agencies.

Everyone would be required to present the card when seeking employment or government benefits, when opening new accounts with financial institutions and in a variety of other circumstances associated with the receipt of income and transfer of funds.

Each organisation would report to central authorities (at this stage only the Tax Office) using the number. The Government asserted that gains would arise in a variety of ways from this arrangement, but offered little explanation of the mechanisms. When challenged by the Joint Select Committee, the Tax Office claimed that their estimates of gains were based on 'qualitative assessment'.

A fuller account and analysis of the Australia Card story may be found in an article by Roger Clarke.[51]

It was apparent from the interviews that this scheme had left a legacy of suspicion and consequently any move towards a centralised national patient record system was regarded as anathema to many Australians.

In spite of this, the General Practice Computing Group brought forward a proposal in 2001 to establish a national electronic prescribing record:[52]

> The proposal which follows is an exciting step in using information technology to bring together our current fragmented medication record systems. It has the potential to assist in achieving significantly better health outcomes for all Australians, by influencing the environment in which prescribing decisions are made, and by promoting informed medication management partnerships between consumers and their doctors and pharmacists.

The proposal is to create a new electronic patient medication record which is put together by linking prescriptions written by different doctors or dispensed by different pharmacists. The contents of such a record are defined in the recommendations in Section 47 of this paper. The medication record is totally accessible to the patient, who has to consent before it can be used by their doctor or pharmacist, and who can include any notes they wish to make and check who has had access to it.

Participation will be voluntary for consumers, prescribers and dispensers, and regulated and monitored by an independent governance body. Nobody will have a new medication record unless they agree. The record is safeguarded by stringent privacy protection and complaints mechanisms.

The electronic patient medication record will be a major advance on our current prescribing systems in Australia, which operate very much at the level of individual prescriptions. There is at present no easy way of putting these records together for an individual. It is particularly difficult for patients on multiple medications, who have to try and remember them all – including strengths, dosage and changes in medication – when they visit other doctors or specialists.

With such a fragmented approach to medication records, there is always a possibility of adverse interactions between medications and inconsistent prescribing by different doctors. One doctor does not know what another has prescribed. The system being proposed here would facilitate the many benefits which can flow from collating all medication information for each individual. An electronic patient medication record is a tool which gives us the chance to achieve big improvements in health outcomes. Consumers can take a much more active and informed part in decisions about their health. Prescribing decisions can be made in the context of full and timely knowledge of a patient's medication history.

Medication details can be entered once, and from then on accessed as needed and agreed by the individual and the doctor or pharmacist they are using. If a person goes to a different doctor or pharmacist, with their agreement that doctor or pharmacist can call up their full medication record.

The electronic patient medication record sets a framework for consumers to enjoy a much safer prescribing and medication management experience. Not only will the danger of misinterpreted handwritten prescriptions be avoided, doctors will no longer have to rely just on their own records for a patient. If they participate in the new arrangements, consumers can go to any doctor knowing that they can make available to that doctor full, accurate and up-to-date information about their current medications, together with information about any previous adverse drug reactions, so that the doctor can prescribe for them safely and confidently. The medication record will also allow consumers to participate in a much more informed way in their partnership with doctors and pharmacists about their healthcare.

This proposal raises many questions about an electronic patient medication record which will need further consideration and consultation.

It has been developed in the considered context of a range of other health policies and initiatives, to ensure that it is consistent with their objectives. These include, among others, the Quality Use of Medicines Policy, decision support initiatives, the National Pharmaceutical Coding Project and the National Electronic Health Records Taskforce. As this proposal is developed in parallel with these important initiatives, it will need to be reviewed and tailored to ensure that it fits in with the broader health information management agenda, particularly the report of the National Electronic Health Records Taskforce regarding the best approach for a national network of electronic health records.

(General Practice Computing Group,
Royal Australian College of GPs)

This proposal does show significant differences from the earlier Australia Card scheme:

- it covers only health, and then only prescribing
- it is voluntary, and includes specific safeguards for patients.

A draft of the proposed Better Medication Management System (BMMS) legislation was forwarded to selected health industry and consumer representatives in May 2001, along with a summary explaining the broad provisions in the bill.[53]

Given that I carried out the interviews in 2001 in the three months following the publication of the draft legislation, and that interviewees frequently raised the issue of privacy, it does suggest that the Government may not have sought a full and frank debate around this initiative.

The legislation is currently (in late 2002) undergoing field testing.

A further issue arising from the independent nature of doctors was the issue of patients receiving treatment simultaneously from a number of GPs. The most extreme case was described to me by a GP:

My patients would come to me for treatment relating to their AIDS or hepatitis. They would visit another GP closer to home for their routine medication, and that physician might not know of their condition.

(GP)

This raised serious issues for me around the balance between confidentiality and the risk to patients' health. Upon return to the UK, I queried this with a UK GP and asked him if the position was similar here. He replied:

If a patient is diagnosed with a condition such as AIDS by an outside agency, for example an STD [sexually transmitted diseases] clinic, that diagnosis would not necessarily be reported to their GP.

(GP)

Whilst this reflects a vital sensitivity to the need for confidentiality around diseases which may carry a significant stigma in society, it undermines the principle that UK GPs have overall responsibility for the care of their patients, and it is possible that this principle is not necessarily carried over to other conditions that may carry equal stigma, e.g. mental health problems.

Hospital doctors commented on the implications of the lack of integrated records:

> I still do a number of clinics in the hospital. A patient may have visited a range of doctors in primary and secondary care. I can spend an hour on the phone trying to confirm a medical history.
>
> (Academic clinician)

The final theme arising from discussions around GPs concerned the introduction of accreditation for GPs.

The accreditation mechanism is known as the Practice Incentives Programme (PIP).[54] It aims to recognise general practices that provide comprehensive, quality care, and which are working towards meeting the Royal Australian College of General Practitioners (RACGP) entry standards for general practices. The PIP is part of a blended payment approach for general practice. Payments made through the Programme are in addition to other income earned by the GPs and the practice, such as patient payments and Medicare rebates.

The PIP aims to compensate for the limitations of fee-for-service arrangements. Under these arrangements, practices that provide numerous quick consultations receive higher rewards than those that take time to look after the ongoing healthcare needs of their patients. High throughput of patients is also associated with unnecessary prescribing, tests and referrals.

PIP payments are dependent on practice size, in terms of patients seen rather than on the number of consultations performed. The additional funding is intended to reduce the pressure on practices to see more patients, more quickly, in order to maximise their income. Since August 1999, payments have focused upon aspects of general practice that contribute to quality care rather than patient continuity.

One of the GPs interviewed was a PIP assessor:

> PIP, which is worth $20 000 to a practice, so ... and that's what everyone has to do, except people who don't want to claim PIP, and they are just stupid. When you sign up, you are given a workbook and the workbook is ... actually you are given a number of things – first you are given a copy of the standards and it is written in very clear, standard language.
>
> I am the only GP I know who has written national standards – that's not true, there are other GPs who have done it – so I know how hard it is to write standards. The national practice standards are actually not bad. So, you are given a copy of the standards and you are also given the reference books that contain the standards so that you just have to follow the cook book – it's not that difficult and if you don't know how to do it, here's the number of the person, you can ring them up. Then you get a workbook – the workbook says start by doing this and then you ought to do this and have you done that and ticked off the item, and you are given a time-line.
>
> ... We took all the stuff and we treated the workbook like a bible – I mean, we did everything we were supposed to do and we actually invented our own package and procedures manual. We sat around in the practice and one receptionist had got this bit and one receptionist

got that bit etc. That is the way it should be so every practice should do it that way. It is a wonderful exercise and if only they understood that – well then that would be against it – you can't teach these people stuff.

These days most practices don't do this – they call up the Division and say 'I can't do this, can you help me please' and the Division goes round and helps them. I say that wearing a forked tongue – why? – because I am one of the people who goes out and earns money.

OK, so they have a lot of, or they should have a lot of, support from their Division. They then book their business and they can either be assessed by a general practitioner with a non-GP or another GP. It is actually faster and cheaper if they have a non-GP because the GP gets paid more than the non-GP. Many of the closed-minded people will only have GPs.

Before we arrive, the practice has to do a patient satisfaction questionnaire. They have to do 100 patients and the questionnaire has to fulfil certain criteria and there is never a questionnaire that isn't perfect, you know. So, I get the checklist to work through and we also get our own workbook that actually has every question that we have to ask all written out so the script is the same for everybody. So, we arrive – we look at the outside of the practice – it's got to be identifiable, it's got to have other various stuff like that.

We then walk in and we agree with our relevant person and we have a little tour of the practice. We note things like – it looks clean, it's been painted, there's no dirt on the floor. We need to make sure that there is a sign for the toilets and that the toilets actually work and that there is water in the tap. We are talking about a very basic level of accreditation. And, as I say, having actually done an accreditation in another practice, the banality of the GP level is frightening except where you have a lot of practices where they haven't got **** all.

We then divide the checks amongst the surveyors. The principal surveyor checks the doctor's bags to make sure there are no out-of-date drugs, and you know you are told all this stuff so if you haven't got it all perfect then you are just a **** basically. That person also checks the notes, which can be very difficult if there are handwritten cards or can be amazingly wonderful if they are computerised.

Meanwhile the accompanying surveyor is talking to the practice manager and to a non-medical member of staff – it can be whoever they want. They ask a whole set of questions which are actually asked to all the same people. We ask the principal doctor, we ask any doctors who are working for the practice, and they ask a member of staff essentially the same sort of things. And they come under a number of standard questions.

They are along the lines of 'How do you do triage?' And they discuss all sorts of treatments, what do you do with people who come to the practice, what happens if people ask for a second opinion, what do you do with dead patients notes, how do you take your notes, how do you keep your notes, how do you maintain confidentiality – all that bull***t and they will ask anybody. And again, they have told you that they are going to ask you all these questions. You then have to go and check the sterilisation excruciatingly and that is potentially always a problem because most people who are doing it, don't know what they are doing. Sometimes people understand what they are doing but a lot of people don't.

Now, again, there is a huge amount of preparation support if you want it. You can buy training and the training is fantastic but again, a lot of doctors don't want to do that. Well, they should do it, because you know if your sterilisation is 'f***ed up'. Alternately, you forget sterilisation and don't do it. Why bother? Checking the vaccine systems, what the processes are for, maintaining them and all that kind of stuff. You also have to check their day book and their health insurance commission outcomes to get evidence that they actually do the visits that they say they do.

When you are looking for a patient, that is generally 25 notes, please, please find one where there is evidence of a phone-call, evidence of a home visit, evidence of an after-hour call. When we did it, we knew they were coming, so we said OK we want that one, that one and that one. Then the two surveyors get together and they pool their two workbooks into a third workbook and we have to work out together.

You could do better, but it's not that important and we are going to let you know that it doesn't matter … so if you actually meet the care and the standards even though it's not the way we thought, that's OK. I surveyed a unique, well, a very strange practice that not only isn't computerised but doesn't have any staff – they have a computer in the waiting room that keeps flashing on – they have no appointments, it is totally walk-in, they have no one to answer the phone, and they actually met a lot of things that we were very worried about. For example, one of the criteria is that there has to be someone else in the practice apart from the doctor at all times. Now they don't because they don't have anyone except the doctors in the practice so they are not going to pass that because that is the way their practice is structured. But they have close circuit television in the waiting room.

But what we do, is we say 'wonderful, wonderful … this is good, this is bad, this is good', something like that. Compliment them on that 'but there are a few things that you really ought to do something about … see how you don't keep copies of your bills at the moment?'

We as assessors have an obligation to be especially nice and helpful. Occasionally we come across a practice that just didn't get the message. One practice sent me a textbook [laughter]. One of the doctors, who is a consultant, knew my name and I had heard of her, and I didn't realise that it was her practice that I was assessing, so I said 'Oh, wow, gosh that's a lot of work' – admire, admire, admire – 'Gee, you know, this is a really interesting practice', and 'One of the things that we have got in my practice is these mobile ramps, the fold-up, fibre-glass ramps which you can put at your front door for wheelchairs. If you've got a practice actually on the street, the council will not allow you to put it out, so one of our patients who is in a wheelchair carried one round and I said where did you get that? It is perfectly wonderful, so I mention this to every practice that I go to who don't have proper wheelchair ramps.' So I mentioned this to her, and so she has this book, this reference book – she says to me thank you so much, it was lovely to have your assessment etc. By the way, can you tell me where to get those ramps. So I was ringing around …

(GP, also a PIP assessor)

The gist of it was that this assessor believed that the standards required were very basic and the financial incentives were very high. Therefore any practice not meeting the standards were 'just stupid'. Whilst the accreditation process might prevent gross problems, it was unlikely to contribute greatly to best practice.

The CEO from the Division of General Practice agrees, albeit a little less colourfully:

That's another little thing that the Government couldn't resist. Who could argue in any defensible manner that their practice shouldn't be a certain standard. Indefensible – not to agree to that. While it is actually the case that they are capturing a number of practices that have languished back there and are bringing them up to a standard.

Now there is no requirement to be accredited – it's not the law, but you can't get any of your PIP payments unless you're an accredited practice from January next year. They have given them two whole years to get accredited – two and a half years. And if you choose not to – that's your independence again – but we are not going to provide you with any incentive payments and most practices, the majority I can't say exactly, are being accredited. And again, it's the profession – a professional is managing it, the Government just supply funding to start the accreditation agency, which has been paid back pretty much now because the doctors pay another GP to do it. And PIP is worth on average somewhere between $10 000 and $20 000 a year per GP so there is a big incentive to get your practice accredited.

(CEO, Division of General Practice)

# The problems of rural populations

One of the key issues facing both Australia and Canada are the problems of rural populations. Both countries have very large areas with very sparse populations. The issue of providing healthcare to rural populations is problematic for the following reasons:

- poor remuneration of physicians
- consequent difficulty in recruitment
- poor access to services for patients
- limited or no choice for patients.

The Commonwealth Government has a range of initiatives designed to improve rural health. They have developed a measure of accessibility and remoteness known as the Australian Remoteness Index (ARIA).[55] The results have been developed as a map, shown in Figure 7.1

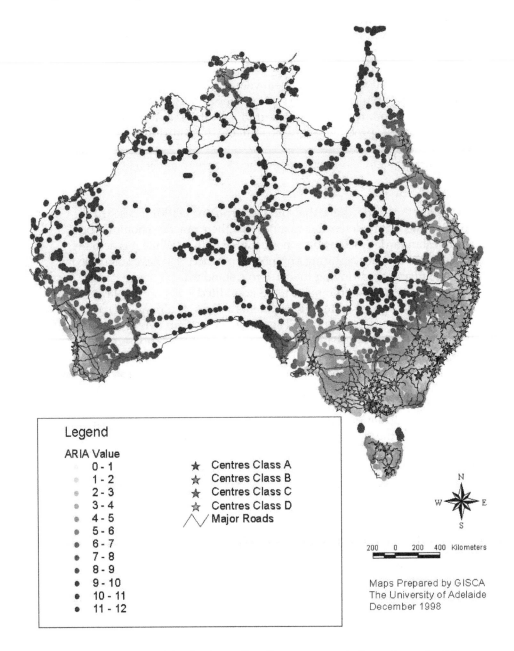

**Figure 7.1** Map produced by the Australian Government to indicate the scale of the problems in terms of remoteness and access to health facilities. See the website for the original colour version.

The map clearly identifies that away from the south east and south west coastal areas, almost all of the landmass of Australia is remote and inaccessible.

In 1911, 43% of Australians lived in rural areas. This proportion fell steadily and in 1976, 14% of the population lived in rural areas. Between 1976 and 1991 the decline appeared to have halted, with a slight increase in the proportion of people living in rural areas (*see* Figure 7.2), which may have been due to people moving to rural areas surrounding the cities, but still working in the city. However, the 1996 Census showed that, once again, the rural population had decreased as a proportion of the total population.

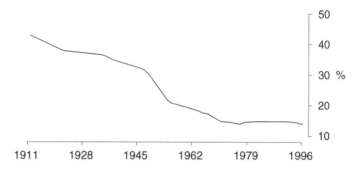

**Figure 7.2**  Rural population, percentage of total population. (Source: ABS data available on request. Census of Population and Housing.)

The Government cites the following initiatives as supporting the delivery of health services in rural areas:

- More doctors for outer metropolitan areas.
- Increased access to Medicare claiming through pharmacies.
- Better treatment for cancer patients in regional areas of Australia Capital.
- Funding boost for rural and regional Australia.
- More aged care nurses for students from regional Australia.
- Additional practice nurses in primary healthcare in areas where patient access to medical services is limited, such as in rural and remote, provincial and outer metropolitan areas with doctor shortages.
- One hundred rural nursing scholarships will be provided for rural students. A further ten scholarships will be available for Aboriginal and Torres Strait Islander nursing students or health workers who want to upgrade their qualifications, funding to develop nine new rural clinical schools and three university departments of rural health, building on the existing university departments of rural health initially funded in the 1996 Budget. These facilities are the foundation of a national rural health education and training network, focusing on providing specific rural health training and encouraging medical and other health professionals to take up rural practice.
- Increasing workforce support for health professionals through the Higher Education Contribution Scheme (HECS). The programme gives graduating medical students the opportunity to 'work off' their HECS debt by taking up employment in rural practice. During 2001–2002 approximately 200 doctors will be assisted under this scheme.

In spite of these measures, there is a need to adopt more radical solutions. One of the solutions being actively pursued in Queensland is the use of telemedicine technology to deliver care to remote areas:

> The big agenda for the Commonwealth is rural access and that is why they are interested in telemedicine. The problem with them is that they are terrified if, in fact, they start funding in the private sector because at the moment it is only funded in the public sector. Under the private sector they have this fantasy that there is going to be this huge cost layout and because it's one man and that there is this unmet need in rural areas in Australia. And you know, somehow some of the Commonwealth bureaucrats believe that doctors are quite prepared to work an extra 24 hours a day to provide a whole lot of new services, which of course they're not. Because what they will actually do is provide services to the bush via video conferencing instead of providing face-to-face services in-house.
>
> I wasn't particularly talking about telemedicine. Australia is well known for it. We do about 2000 hours a month in Queensland, which is very significant. About 70% of that is educational and about 30% is clinical and they keep all data on that. You know, we've got published outcomes – we have just got the latest paper on the last four years of data. It is at the press at the moment but will be published fairly shortly. But we – and Queensland Health is using some of this quality money – are using about $1m in telemedicine to essentially try and develop it in a strategic way across the State. So the term telemedicine is generally used.
>
> Australia is constantly mentioned in all the documents and it is politically flash. The systems are used quite heavily, which is good but they are not used to the extent that they should be. When you look at the overall number of consultations, the numbers aren't huge in telemedicine. So as I say, it has been used more educationally. We are trying to reverse that and one of the interesting projects that we are doing with that is again a human issue; it's not a technology issue, it's not just a technology process.
>
> We've a very good project going at the moment through children's hospitals here whereby we have set up an internal electronic triage that is a human triage system basically, so that if you're phoning and you want an appointment for any reason as a GP for any of your patients, and you come from a couple of areas of the State, then you just ring a single phone number and you get to speak to an experienced triage nurse who will then go and physically find a consultant and get that consultant to either ring you, email you or make a conference with you and see you or your patient depending on what is necessary in your home town. They can make a decision with you as to whether that patient needs to be referred down here or transferred here or whatever. And so what we have done is set up a one-stop internal referral system which is essentially a phone-call, a call centre, except it's run by a nurse who knows everyone and who is able to check to make sure that they actually do consult back quickly with the GP and that sort of thing. It is a very interesting model.

It's a model that the hospital is really pleased about and I think we will probably be inclined to work it through our whole system. I can easily imagine that we will have four or five nurses working across the hospital providing essentially an electronic triage service for all the services – you know, for out-patients and for all non walk-in emergencies. And that to me is actually a very good way of going, and then we will be using our 200 video conferencing units around the State, so there is a huge network available. We can essentially video-conference to anywhere in the State and we will cover the east coast, of which there are 28 hospitals, over the next 18 months, so we will have broadband available in all hospitals. We have that process of a clinical triage system in the major hospitals and the ability to then get back in the broadband immediately to local areas. And that, I think, is actually a really nice model and would work really well in the UK. I think it's a really good way of using tertiary centres in particular. It is dependent on essentially the ability to have good quality triage people who are clinicians and who can then grab the right consultant or whoever to talk to for a referral. It's looking really good at the moment.

(Academic clinician)

The issues about embedding this kind of hi-tech solution into the healthcare system appears to be well advanced:

As regarding quality generally, I mean, in telemedicine there is a national telehealth committee … so telehealth has come very much from the national agenda through that process. It's always assumed ultimately that telehealth will disappear and will just become parallel with the healthcare. I think it should disappear. We now talk about e-health or on-line health as being an ordinary term and you know you're either seeing people face to face or you're seeing them electronically.

(Academic clinician)

There are other initiatives to provide better coverage and choice for rural populations. For example:

I work in a scheme to visit rural communities and provide a female GP in areas. We go in and run clinics in communities where only male GPs are usually available.

(Urban female GP)

However, other pressures are reducing the ability of GPs to meet the needs of their patients:

Traditionally, the country GP would deliver the vast majority of babies in rural communities. Now the cost of indemnity insurance makes this impossible. Whilst this is alleged to protect women by ensuring that their births are overseen by a specialist, it also entails an inconvenient and potentially hazardous journey for otherwise healthy mothers and babies.

(CEO, Division of General Practice)

# Conclusions

## Are the policy values carried into practice?

The Australian policy documents emphasise that the system is effectively a private insurance system regulated by the public sector. The purpose of this is to provide a degree of patient choice at reasonable cost. It necessitates a system of accreditation in order to regulate the private elements of the system.

The most successful part of this is the provision of a system based upon patient choice. At least in the urban centres Australian patients have a high degree of choice when compared with their UK counterpart, and access to care is generally much better.

The other objective of reasonable cost is more questionable. Estimates suggest that the Australian Federal Government has spent $800m Au. in promoting the uptake of private healthcare with little benefit in outcomes and waiting times. Further, some of the schemes around lifetime guarantees over premiums have implications for future costs.

The use of accreditation systems and indicators is also limited in its success. Accreditation in hospitals is well established and appears to work reasonably well. In primary care, there was more cynicism over the system and it appears to be of more limited value.

## Strengths, weaknesses, opportunities and threats in healthcare in Australia

The study has revealed the following SWOTs (*see* Box 7.1).

---

**Box 7.1** SWOTs in healthcare in Australia

*Strengths*
- Patient choice
- Access to care
- Commitment to universality

*Weaknesses*
- Cost of promoting private care
- Cost of private provision of public provision
- Lack of choice in rural areas

*Opportunities*
- Telehealth in rural areas
- Establishment of national electronic prescribing records

*Threats*
- Commercial conflicts of interests
- Litigation and costs of indemnity insurance
- Vulnerability of commercial insurers and healthcare providers

---

The Australian Government has spent significant sums in increasing the uptake of private healthcare insurance. There is little evidence that this has been effective in improving outcomes and reducing waiting times in the public system. On the other hand, Australian patients, or at least that subsection that can access private services, value the choice that their system provides.

One of the most startling paradoxes is the proud independence of GPs and their defence of the patient's right to choose their primary care set alongside the rush to sell out to the corporate players.

# CHAPTER 8

# What is the reality in Canada?

## Historical development

Undoubtedly, the most significant development in the history of healthcare in Canada was the introduction of the Canada Health Act.

The first step towards universal public coverage began with the introduction of hospitalisation insurance in Saskatchewan in 1947. Then, in 1957, the Federal Government committed to sharing the costs of hospitalisation insurance with the provinces. This financial assistance encouraged the eventual creation of similar Medicare programmes in all provinces by 1961. It quickly became apparent that if the goal was to protect Canadians' health, then it made sense to extend public funding beyond hospitalisation insurance to include family physicians.

Two quite different approaches were proposed:

- a multi-payer system that encouraged Canadians to purchase the private insurance of their choice (or pay out of pocket if they chose not to buy any insurance), while providing some public coverage to the poorest in society
- a single-payer system that provided universal coverage to everyone on the same basis (without out-of-pocket user payments) and was funded through the tax system.

The debate among healthcare providers, policy experts and governments about the two options was fierce. The public was both torn and confused by the controversy. In 1964, a Commission on Health Services, chaired by Justice Emmett Hall, rejected the multi-payer approach in favour of a single-payer system primarily for two reasons: it was less expensive and people with poor health and those who were less well off would be better served.

It would take another eight years and considerable debate for the Hall Commission recommendations to be implemented, and almost 20 years before the Canada Health Act gave them the full authority of legislation.[56]

1961: Conservative Prime Minister John Diefenbaker appoints Supreme Court Justice Emmett Hall to head the Emmett Hall Commission on Health Services.

1962: CCF Premier Woodrow Lloyd extends universal, publicly financed insurance to physician services in Saskatchewan. This is followed by a doctors' strike that lasts 23 days.

1964: Emmett Hall's report recommends publicly funded, universal insurance, not only for doctors' services, but also for prescription drugs and home care, as well as dental and optical services for some groups.

1966: Prime Minister Lester Pearson's Liberal Government introduces the Medical Care Act – quickly to become known as 'Medicare'.

1968–1972: Through an intense series of intergovernmental negotiations, all ten provinces and two territories eventually 'sign on' to Medicare, agreeing to provide universal public coverage for hospital and physician care in exchange for federal contributions towards the costs.

In the 1960s and 1970s, all provinces eventually dropped a private insurance model in favour of a public model. The majority of Canadians eventually concluded that a public model better reflected the value of equitable and unimpeded access to necessary hospital and physician services by tying access to need rather than ability to pay.

In 1985, mainly in response to a simmering dispute over extra billing (charging patients in excess of the rates covered by public insurance), Parliament passed the Canada Health Act[57] and, for the first time, some of the motivating principles behind national Medicare were made explicit.

As an outsider in Canada, I observe that to many Canadians this Act has achieved the same status as the Constitution in the United States. In view of its crucial nature and its unique status in Canadian healthcare policy development, we shall consider it in some detail. Box 8.1 contains its key passages.

Coming to this document as an outsider, the first thing that strikes me is that the Act actually explicitly states the values upon which the Act is based. In that sense, it may be seen as strongly the fundamental hypothesis on which this whole book is based, i.e. that our healthcare systems are based upon a set of values, normally implicit, but explicit in the Canada Health Act.

The second observation would be that the Act derives its authority from both popular will and hard economics. The Act reflects that at least in 1985, the battle for the values espoused by Emmett Hall had been won. At the same time, the mechanism for implementation is based upon hard economics within the federal/provincial split. The provinces are not required to follow the model, simply that if they do not follow the model, funding will not be supplied from the Federal Government.

The five criteria have assumed huge importance in any discussion on what a good healthcare system should provide in Canada. However, there is significant flexibility in how to interpret the meaning of the principles and they also have some inherent limitations, which have become more apparent as the health agenda has developed since the 1960s.

First, the Canada Health Act covers only hospital and physician services. Innovations in treatment, like preventive health programmes and community-based initiatives, are not generally covered, nor are home care, long-term care, dental care or prescription drug therapies (unless provided in hospitals). The hard evidence for this comes from the percentage of health expenditure coming from the public sector. The percentage of health expenditure from the public sector in Canada is no greater than the percentage in the Australian system, which proudly boasts of its private healthcare system and is less than that of the UK.

**Box 8.1**   Key passages of the Canada Health Act[57]

In order that a province may qualify for a full cash contribution referred to in section 5 for a fiscal year, the healthcare insurance plan of the province must, throughout the fiscal year, satisfy the criteria described in sections 8 to 12 respecting the following matters:

(a) public administration
(b) comprehensiveness
(c) universality
(d) portability
(e) accessibility.

8 Public administration
8 (1) In order to satisfy the criterion respecting public administration:
　　(a) the healthcare insurance plan of a province must be administered and operated on a non-profit basis by a public authority appointed or designated by the government of the province;
　　(b) the public authority must be responsible to the provincial government for that administration and operation; and
　　(c) the public authority must be subject to audit of its accounts and financial transactions by such authority as is charged by law with the audit of the accounts of the province.

Designation of agency permitted:
　(2) The criterion respecting public administration is not contravened by reason only that the public authority referred to in subsection (1) has the power to designate any agency:
　　(a) to receive on its behalf any amounts payable under the provincial healthcare insurance plan; or
　　(b) to carry out on its behalf any responsibility in connection with the receipt or payment of accounts rendered for insured health services, if it is a condition of the designation that all those accounts are subject to assessment and approval by the public authority and that the public authority shall determine the amounts to be paid in respect thereof.

9 Comprehensiveness
**9** In order to satisfy the criterion respecting comprehensiveness, the healthcare insurance plan of a province must insure all insured health services provided by hospitals, medical practitioners or dentists, and where the law of the province so permits, similar or additional services rendered by other healthcare practitioners.

10 Universality

**10** In order to satisfy the criterion respecting universality, the healthcare insurance plan of a province must entitle one hundred per cent of the insured persons of the province to the insured health services provided for by the plan on uniform terms and conditions.

11 Portability

**11** (1) In order to satisfy the criterion respecting portability, the healthcare insurance plan of a province:

    (a) must not impose any minimum period of residence in the province, or waiting period, in excess of three months before residents of the province are eligible for or entitled to insured health services;

    (b) must provide for and be administered and operated so as to provide for the payment of amounts for the cost of insured health services provided to insured persons while temporarily absent from the province on the basis that:

        (i) where the insured health services are provided in Canada, payment for health services is at the rate that is approved by the healthcare insurance plan of the province in which the services are provided, unless the provinces concerned agree to apportion the cost between them in a different manner, or

        (ii) where the insured health services are provided out of Canada, payment is made on the basis of the amount that would have been paid by the province for similar services rendered in the province, with due regard, in the case of hospital services, to the size of the hospital, standards of service and other relevant factors; and

    (c) must provide for and be administered and operated so as to provide for the payment, during any minimum period of residence, or any waiting period, imposed by the healthcare insurance plan of another province, of the cost of insured health services provided to persons who have ceased to be insured persons by reason of having become residents of that other province, on the same basis as though they had not ceased to be residents of the province.

Requirement for consent for elective insured health services permitted:

(2) The criterion respecting portability is not contravened by a requirement of a provincial healthcare insurance plan that the prior consent of the public authority that administers and operates the plan must be obtained for elective insured health services provided to a resident of the province while temporarily absent from the province if the services in question were available on a substantially similar basis in the province.

12 Accessibility

**12** (1) In order to satisfy the criterion respecting accessibility, the healthcare insurance plan of a province:

> (a) must provide for insured health services on uniform terms and conditions and on a basis that does not impede or preclude, either directly or indirectly whether by charges made to insured persons or otherwise, reasonable access to those services by insured persons;
>
> (b) must provide for payment for insured health services in accordance with a tariff or system of payment authorized by the law of the province;
>
> (c) must provide for reasonable compensation for all insured health services rendered by medical practitioners or dentists; and
>
> (d) must provide for the payment of amounts to hospitals, including hospitals owned or operated by Canada, in respect of the cost of insured health services.

Reasonable compensation:

> (2) In respect of any province in which extra billing is not permitted, paragraph (1)(c) shall be deemed to be complied with if the province has chosen to enter into, and has entered into, an agreement with the medical practitioners and dentists of the province that provides:
>
> (a) for negotiations relating to compensation for insured health services between the province and provincial organizations that represent practising medical practitioners or dentists in the province;
>
> (b) for the settlement of disputes relating to compensation through, at the option of the appropriate provincial organizations referred to in paragraph (a), conciliation or binding arbitration by a panel that is equally representative of the provincial organizations and the province and that has an independent chairman; and
>
> (c) that a decision of a panel referred to in paragraph (b) may not be altered except by an Act of the legislature of the province.

The reason for this is that the Canadian system is essentially binary in nature: whilst the majority of services are covered 100% by the public sector, those that aren't are entirely private. In Australia, most services are a public–private mix. Also, in the Canadian system, two of the areas not covered by Medicare – drugs outside hospital and long-term care – are significant and growing areas of expenditure.

Second, there is genuine disagreement over how to interpret these broad principles and what is meant by terms such as 'medically necessary' or 'accessibility'. At the 2002 Canadian Health Economics Research Association (CHERA) conference, Charles Wright addressed this issue head on:

> I have the greatest respect for Justice Hall, but he had one very serious flaw which is unfortunately shared by all of us, namely he was completely unable to see clearly 40 years in the future. Working in the early

1960s, he was focused on providing 'medically necessary services' to sick people. We are now into a healthcare system that goes way beyond that mandate to an extent that could not have been imagined. In addition to providing care for people that Justice Hall recognized as being ill, we are now providing a wide range of services in disease prevention, health promotion and screening for disease. Many drugs and operations are dealing with the diseases associated with the ageing process that simply had to be tolerated in the past.

The medicalization of the human condition has reached an incredible level that is now almost certainly crossing the border between net benefit and harm.

(Emmett Hall Memorial Lecture, CHERA 2002)[58]

The implicit message is that, without cost as a controlling mechanism, demand in a publicly funded system will grow infinitely. Interestingly, my UK-centric conclusion, from the observation that the Canadian healthcare system has become over-medicalised, is that there is a need to improve screening and prevention, but this gets short shrift here. Breast and prostate screening are lumped in with the overuse of antibiotics in children and the rapid growth in elective Caesarean sections.

Also from a UK-centric perspective, it is refreshing to hear a debate about over-provision of service within a public system, rather than the constant debate over how much more we need to provide to meet basic needs.

The different interpretation of these principles comes to the fore most obviously in disputes between the Federal and provincial governments.

Under the Canadian system, the Federal Government is responsible for:

- setting and administering national principles or standards for the healthcare system (for example, through the Canada Health Act)
- assisting in the financing of provincial healthcare services through fiscal transfers
- delivering direct health services to specific groups, including veterans, native Canadians, people living on reserves, military personnel, inmates of federal penitentiaries and the Royal Canadian Mounted Police
- fulfilling other health-related functions, such as health protection, disease prevention and health promotion.

The provincial and territorial governments are responsible for:

- managing and delivering health services
- planning, financing and evaluating the provision of hospital care and physician and allied healthcare services
- managing some aspects of prescription care and public health.

This leaves the provinces in Canada in a much stronger position that the States in Australia. There are significant differences among the provinces in terms of how they individually understand and apply the principles. However, the Federal Government has the final responsibility for interpreting the Canada Health Act.

For example, the prohibition on extra billing under the Canada Health Act is interpreted by some as absolute and by others as only a limit on the extent of the practice. Because of this type of disagreement over interpretation, there have been calls to revisit the Canada Health Act with a view to establishing new mechanisms or approaches for resolving disputes, rather than leaving decisions solely in the hands of the Federal Government.

The reality is that the Canada Health Act derives its status from being a national piece of legislation. A Health Act interpreted by the provinces is no longer a *Canada* Health Act, but a set of provincial pieces of legislation.

Currently, Canadians have 100% coverage for a core set of hospital, physician and some directly related services that are defined as medically necessary. The assumption behind this policy is that it is more important to cover the most urgent, essential and costly services, rather than those that are considered less necessary. As a result, there are only minor variations across the country in terms of the types of services covered by the Canada Health Act.

This in itself has been challenged by people like Charles Wright, who argue that coverage is now too wide and can no longer be considered to be restricted to 'medically necessary hospital and doctor services'. At the same time, some authors have argued that without Medicare encompassing a comprehensive Pharmacare programme, the coverage is inadequate:[59]

> The National Forum on Health believes that the way to improve appropriate access to and utilization of drugs, and to control the growth of drug expenditures, is to ensure that medically necessary prescription drugs are made available to all Canadian residents, without deductibles or co-payments. International experience has shown that this is best accomplished under a publicly financed and regulated system, which in Canada would, of course, be administered by the provinces with arrangements for portability of benefits – within reasonable constraints – throughout the country. In essence, that requires finding a mechanism to transfer private health expenditures to governments so that they can be managed publicly.
>
> This is the ideal the Forum advocates for the long term. Because financing issues are intrinsically tied to the organization of the health system, and because the organization of our health system is in flux, we can only go so far as to recommend the characteristics of the system that will promote improved management of pharmaceuticals. It will be the responsibility of Federal and provincial governments to establish financial and other incentives that will direct and synchronize reforms across the country. Our proposals should be seen as incremental and interdependent: each requiring political will, financial backing, and persuasive leadership. As a first step toward improving access, we need better information to monitor and evaluate utilization at the individual level, and to facilitate decision making at Federal and provincial levels.
>
> (Final Report of the National Forum on Health, Volume II)

Another area of contention and variation in provincial practice is home care. While all provinces and territories cover professional services such as nursing care, some also provide personal care and homemaking. Some provide meals, home management and maintenance programmes while others do not, and some provide respite and palliative care in the home while others do not. Home care programmes not only vary across the provinces, there also can be variations within provinces in the types of services provided in different health regions and communities. Interestingly, this is one service under local control in the UK where there is significant variation as well. For example, Scotland provides more generous public support than does England or Wales.

The question of how to pay for these additional services is an important one; if the scope of what is covered is broadened, the costs to public treasuries will increase in the short run even if total healthcare costs decline in the long run.

The answer to this issue is not as simple as the Australian Minister of Health would wish to make it. The evidence that we may be able to have at least some cake and eat it is as follows:

- There is evidence that public provision, particularly in the Canadian context, is cheaper than private provision.
- There is some evidence that the cost of healthcare is dominated by the cost of care in the last months of life and that this remains true even as life gets longer.
- There is evidence that increasing drug costs in some cases may be more than offset by savings elsewhere in the system.

However, in the short term in expenditure, the inability to be able to show how increased costs in one part of the system lead to saving elsewhere because of disjointed accounting, and the headline increase in the public expenditure, means that this is a 'brave' option for any politician to pursue.

In the final report of the Romanow Commission on the Future of Healthcare in Canada,[60] published in November 2002, two of the key recommendations relate to drugs and home care:

> *Revise the Canada Health Act to include coverage for home care services in priority areas.*
> Home care is an increasingly essential part of our healthcare system. While it is not possible to include all home care services under the Canada Health Act, immediate steps should be taken to bring services in three priority areas under the umbrella of the Canada Health Act – home mental health case management and intervention services, post-acute home care and palliative home care.
> *Improve the quality of care and support available to people with mental illnesses by including home mental health case management and intervention services as part of the Canada Health Act.*
> Mental health has been described as the 'orphan child' of healthcare. Today, mental healthcare is largely a home- and community-based service, but support for it has too frequently fallen short. It is time to take the long overdue step of ensuring that mental health home care services are included as medically necessary services under the Canada Health Act, and available across the country.
> *Expand the Canada Health Act to include coverage for post-acute home care, including medication management and rehabilitation services.*
> Advances in medical technologies and treatments mean that many procedures that previously required long hospital stays can be replaced by day surgeries or brief overnight stays. But many patients still need

follow-up care and rehabilitation services in their own home. Providing coverage for post-acute home care services across the country on equal terms and conditions through the Canada Health Act is a necessary and logical next step. Coverage for post-acute home care should include case management, health professional services and medication management.

(p.xxxi)

However, the report recognises financial realities and neither the home care nor drug reforms amounts to a whole-scale reform:[60]

Because of the significant costs that would be involved in including all home care services under the Canada Health Act, priorities should be placed on the most pressing needs. There is little doubt that effective home care support is vitally important to people with mental illnesses, to people who have just been released from hospital and to those who are in their last months of life. These three areas – mental health, post-acute care and palliative care – should be the first three home care services to be included under a revised Canada Health Act.

(p.172)

Given the expanding role of prescription drugs in Canada's healthcare system, a strong case can be made that prescription drugs are just as medically necessary as hospital or physician services (National Forum on Health, 1997). However, the immediate integration of all prescription drugs into a revised Canada Health Act has significant implications, not the least of which would be substantial costs. Therefore, the goal should be to move in a gradual but deliberate and dedicated way to integrate prescription drugs more fully into the continuum of care. Over time, these proposals will raise the floor for prescription drug coverage across Canada and lay the groundwork for the ultimate objective of bringing prescription drugs under the Canada Health Act.

(p.190)

# What the people say

Interviews took place with a similar range of personnel as in Australia, from two provinces, Ontario and Alberta. Constraints upon time meant fewer interviews with practitioners. As far as possible, this was compensated for by attendance at a number of health service research conferences, which provided the opportunity to meet with many researchers from across Canada, who in turn referred me to much of their own evidence. Informal conversations with patients drew on their experiences from a wider range of provinces. The themes emerging from the conversations were:

- the role of doctors
- the role of private healthcare
- the role of primary care.

# The role of doctors

The views expressed about doctors in the UK were echoed in Canada:

> Doctors are overpaid and far too powerful in the Canadian system. I used to have some good friends as doctors and we used to go hill-walking together, but I realised that we'd moved apart when their idea of a hill-walk was hiring a helicopter to drop them at the top to then walk down! However, most people would exclude their own physician from these criticisms.
>
> (Academic)

Or as a cardiac consultant, who had left the UK NHS to work in the Canadian system, put it:

> The Canadian healthcare system is going down the pan.

**AG**: How bad is it? Are you tempted to go back to the NHS?

> Good God, no, it's not that bad!
>
> (Cardiac consultant)

The emphasis upon 'medically necessary services' in the Canada Health Act has reinforced the historical dominance of the medical profession. Nurse practitioners are still relatively uncommon and the nursing profession in general has less status in Canada than the UK. Midwives have only been part of the Medicare system since 1994 in Ontario.

An expectant father from Alberta was appalled at the idea of a midwife-led delivery:

> I think it's terrible. I can't imagine having a birth where the doctor wasn't present and in charge. It seems such a terrible risk to take.

In Alberta, midwives are not covered by the Alberta Health Insurance Plan.[61] In British Columbia, midwives have been allowed to practice since 1998 and there are now some 88 midwives registered in the province. However, only deliveries supervised by physicians are eligible for reimbursement, although physicians can bill for midwifery services.

This much lower profile for midwives, compared to the UK, is mirrored in Australia where there are approximately 7000 midwives. However, they have been almost removed from responsibility in the birthing process itself by the withdrawal of indemnity insurance, in common with GPs.[62]

We shall return to the theme of the dominant position of physicians when we consider primary care and its reform.

# The role of private healthcare

It has often been stated to the author that there is no private healthcare in Canada. In practice, this means that private healthcare providers do not duplicate the services provided under the Canada Health Act in the way that in the UK private providers duplicate the services provided by the NHS.

Some respondents expressed the view that a mixed private–public model would inevitably lead to a reduction in the quality of the public system and an increase in costs:

> There will never be a high-quality public system in the UK whilst you permit private healthcare.
>
> (Manager)

> There is plenty of evidence that private provision would increase costs. The current pressure to allow more private care in Canada makes no sense. The only excuse for doing it would be to shift costs around within the system.
>
> (Academic)

Other voices were more cynical:

> There is private healthcare for Canadians. Those who want private care simply go over the border to the States.
>
> (Doctor)

Even within Canada, provincial variations in interpreting the Canada Health Act lead to accusations that some provinces are in breach of the Act:

> There are many clinics in Alberta effectively carrying out private care and infringing the Act.
>
> (Academic, from outside Alberta)

> Clinics were established to carry out procedures not covered by the scope of the Act. Gradually, they have been drawn into the delivery of care under the Act.
>
> (Academic clinician, Alberta)

It is necessary to distinguish between the private delivery of healthcare paid for by public schemes and private delivery of healthcare paid for privately by the patient either directly or through insurance. One interviewee drew my attention to comments from Wendy Armstrong of the Consumer Association of Canada, Alberta branch, who stated that:

> The real problem we have found in Alberta with our over 50 private, investor-owned day surgery clinics is that private delivery and private payment ultimately walk hand in hand because they really aren't more efficient or cheaper unless they provide less or charge more on top of the public reimbursement. It also has become pretty apparent that privatization walks hand in hand with commercialization. It appears that you can't give the responsibility to deliver medical care to commercial interests and not expect them to adopt all the commercial trappings, including aggressive marketing, focus on increased sales and pursuit of returns (profit). In such an environment, even the community-controlled facilities start taking on these values.

There is a clear division between those who believe that the system must be public in its entirety and those who believe that private organisations can bring efficiency savings to the public system. The first expresses a value that healthcare should be owned by all for the good of all and that it is ethically wrong to make money out of someone else's illness. The second is more pragmatic and believes that private delivery is necessarily more expensive.

Even Professor Bob Evans, an eloquent and vocal champion of public Medicare, who described the idea of private healthcare delivery being cheaper as:

> like a zombie. Every time you knock it down with the evidence, it keeps coming back. You can't kill it because it's never really alive.[12]

admits that:

> From the outset, however, it is important to emphasize that profit *per se* is associated with neither moral turpitude nor additional costs.[63]

Professor Raisa Deber, in her discussion paper for the Romanow Commission, provides one of the best discussions of these issues.[64] The highlights of the arguments are:

- How care is financed is not the same as how it is delivered.
- 'Private delivery' is not a homogeneous category. Private providers can be not-for-profit (NFP) or for-profit (FP); in turn, for-profit includes a range from small businesses (FP/s), such as physicians' offices, to corporate organisations which are expected to provide returns on investment to their shareholders (FP/c). The characteristics and implications of these different types of organisations vary considerably.
- In Canada, most healthcare delivery is already private. Although about 70% of Canadian healthcare is financed publicly, almost all of this care is already delivered by private (usually NFP) providers.
- Comparing public, NFP and FP delivery is complicated because they usually do not offer the same services. Because they need to make a profit, FP organisations will tend to serve potentially profitable services and client groups. Many attempts to compare costs or outcomes are, in effect, comparing 'apples to oranges'.
- The desirability of encouraging FP delivery depends upon how such firms make their profits. Potential 'win–win' situations exist if savings result from strong economies of scale (especially for services which can span jurisdictional boundaries) or better management.
- However, savings frequently arise from more contentious measures, including freedom from labour agreements (and different wage levels and skill mixes), evasion of cost controls placed on other providers, sacrifice of difficult-to-measure intangibles, risk selection/cream skimming or even dubious practices.
- When services are delivered privately, it is necessary to monitor performance. Such monitoring is often costly and difficult; these costs must be included in any fair comparison of alternative delivery approaches.
- Performance monitoring is more likely to work for services whose outcomes are easy to measure; however, many healthcare services are too complex to be treated in this way.

- If performance cannot easily be monitored, NFP delivery is more likely to provide high-quality outcomes than is FP delivery, with FP/c being the most vulnerable to poor outcomes.
- To the extent that economic advantages arise from private delivery, the literature suggests these derive more from the imposition of competition than from ownership type.
- Competition implies low barriers to market entry and exit, and may clash with expertise, trust and cooperation.
- The assumption that we can have a competitive model with a single public payer is naive; firms require either predictable revenue streams or the possibility of revenue generation outside the publicly funded system.
- Experiments should not be irreversible, particularly given international trade agreements.
- Regardless of what decisions are made about delivery, it is essential that the client focus of the existing system be addressed with some urgency to discover why existing NFP organisations appear to be less nimble, innovative and flexible than their FP counterparts.

One of these points was emphasised to me by interviewees:

> In practice, most of the Canadian healthcare is privately delivered. However, most of this is either by not-for-profit or by individual doctors. People here seem reluctant to see people making a profit out of healthcare.

I will use home care in Ontario as a specific example. Home care beyond 'essential medical services' is not covered by the Canada Health Act.

Home care is a growth area of healthcare, partly due to the ageing population and partly due to cost containment. Across Canada, 15 000 nursing positions were eliminated in hospitals from 1990 to 1996, with over half of those being from Ontario hospitals.

In all 12 jurisdictions, the Ministries or Departments of Health and/or Social/Community Services have maintained control over home care budgets and funding levels. Quebec, Prince Edward Island, Northwest Territories and Yukon have Departments of Health and Social Services responsible for home care. Newfoundland and New Brunswick have Departments of Health and Community Services which administer their home care programmes. The remaining six provinces (i.e. British Columbia, Alberta, Saskatchewan, Manitoba, Ontario and Nova Scotia) include home care programmes under the Ministries or Departments of Health.

Most provinces have delegated responsibility for funding allocation and service delivery to regional or local health authorities. However, in most cases the provincial and territorial departments set overall policy guidelines and standards for regional service delivery, reporting requirements and monitoring outcomes.

In recent years, in response to a cost-containment agenda, there has been a trend for provinces to allocate health funds using a population needs-based funding model. Funding levels are determined by population needs-based characteristics rather than on past service use. Another trend that is just beginning is for provinces or regional health authorities to specify that community health budgets cannot be reduced, while hospital acute care and institutional supportive budgets can be decreased to provide additional funding for community budgets.

In Ontario, a new vendor selection system was set up, requiring agencies to compete on the basis of both cost and quality, and opening the door to greater participation by for-profit agencies.

Within Ontario, home care is now administered through Community Care Access Centres. There are 43 Community Care Access Centres (CCACs) in Ontario, two of which are hospital based. CCACs provide a simplified point of access to long-term care for more than 400 000 people each year.

The official information[65] states that the role of CCACs is to:

- arrange and authorise visiting health and personal support services in peoples' homes
- authorise services for special needs children in schools
- manage admissions to long-term care facilities
- provide information and referrals to the public about other community agencies and services.

CCACs are entirely funded by the Ministry of Health and Long-term Care. Services arranged through CCACs include nursing, physiotherapy, occupational therapy, speech and language pathology, dietetic services, social work, personal support and homemaking.

Services are provided on a short-term basis to help people returning home from hospital or recovering from an illness or accident; services are also available on a long-term basis to assist people with disabilities or chronic health problems and to provide palliative care for the terminally ill.

Each CCAC is required to establish a Community Advisory Council to improve integration with local community support agencies, long-term care facilities and hospitals. This improved integration is intended to promote more seamless delivery of services.

They offer a single-entry service point and are responsible for placement in all long-term care facilities, coordinated service planning and monitoring, and case management. CCACs assess need, determine eligibility and purchase services. CCACs have purchased all services since the year 2000, except for assessment, case management, evaluation and monitoring. Following referral, a multi-dimensional assessment of needs and available informal supports is completed, treatment goals are set and a service plan is developed. Case managers are then assigned to coordinate the delivery of home healthcare and homemaking services by various providers according to the client's assessed need for these services. Adults with physical disabilities can access attendant services directly without going through the CCAC.

There is no charge for nursing, therapy, social work, personal support and homemaking services provided through CCACs for persons with assessed service needs up to specified maximums. Persons who wish more services than those for which they have been assessed may purchase them privately. The client is eligible for a drug card which covers drugs related to the admission to the Home Care programme according to provincial formulary. CCACs provide some specified supplies and equipment to support the service plan where appropriate. They do not provide any supplies/equipment that can be made available through Ontario's Assistive Services programme.

CCACs are delivering publicly funded care, albeit funded at a provincial level rather than through Federal funds under the Canada Health Act. However, they have been converted from independent community boards to statutory corporations that comply with Ministry policies, directives and guidelines. CCAC executive directors and board members are appointed by Order in Council. Many regard this with suspicion:

> The new bodies have to drive down costs. They either have to save money on patients or staff. The working conditions for nurses working in the new services have been degraded. Much of the work has been shifted from nurses to care assistants, who are often immigrants who are very badly paid.
>
> (Ex-hospital manager, now independent consultant)

During the transition to the new arrangements there were several strikes over wages and benefits, principally mileage reimbursement for nurses travelling from patient to patient, which were said to be the result of the new competitive bidding process for home care contracts.

In one strike, registered practical nurses in Ontario settled a two-week strike when they accepted an agreement reducing mileage reimbursement from 28–30 cents per kilometre to 17–20 cents per kilometre, a two-year wage freeze, loss of some statutory holidays, decreased vacation pay for part-time and casual nurses, and a drop in employer contributions to health and dental benefits.

For many of the people interviewed, this represents the unacceptable face of private operation within a public system, and sits uncomfortably within the public ethos of the system. In the UK, the trade unions in 2002 have recently made protest over the degradation of staff working conditions by the use of private services within NHS hospitals. Whilst public hospitals have contracted out services for many years, whole hospitals are now being handed over to private management and funding through the Private Finance Initiative. At the time of writing, 63 hospitals are earmarked as PFI projects, with more to follow. In October 2002, the UK government agreed that employees would remain as NHS employees. It means that they retain their pensions and terms and conditions of service, as well as a degree of job security.

There are implications for patients as well. Many existing agencies or networks of nurses established to bid for the work they were already doing had been focused upon delivery of care and did not have expertise in business planning or in competitive tendering:

> They didn't have a clue how to put their bid together. When the result was announced, the existing care providers did not get the contract. The feedback said it was a quality issue. The existing agency hadn't had a complaint in five years. The only quality issue was the quality of the bid itself, not the quality of care.

> When a care provider comes in, many long-term relationships between carers and clients are disrupted. This can leave vulnerable and elderly people confused and unhappy.
>
> (Ex-hospital manager, now independent consultant)

The other area of care highlighted by the Romanow Commission as being strongly privatised within some provinces is the area of diagnostic clinics:[60]

> The growing reliance on private advanced diagnostic services is erod-ing the equal access principle at the heart of Medicare. The CHA must include public coverage for medically necessary diagnostic services. Governments have a responsibility to invest sufficiently in the public system to make timely access to diagnostic services for all a reality. In a similar vein, they should also reconsider the current practice by which some workers' compensation agencies contract with private providers to deliver fast-track diagnostic services to potential claimants.
>
> (p.xxv)

Whether the recommendations in this area can be implemented against the strong vested interests, especially in provinces such as Alberta, remains to be seen.

## The role of primary care

The Canadian system has a tradition of general practice as in the UK and Australia. GP remuneration is based upon fee-for-service, and like Australia, and unlike the UK, patients can visit the doctor of their choice.

From the viewpoint of patients, the fee-for-service remuneration scheme is that it places no significant restrictions on their choice and doctors have an incentive to provide all 'medically necessary services':

> A Canadian GP consultation will be considerably longer than that in the UK, and the doctor will carry out a range of procedures such as blood pressure as a matter of routine.
>
> (Academic clinician)

Thus, in most cases, this leaves patients and doctors happy. Patients feel that they are receiving the care that they need and doctors can bill for their services to reflect the work carried out. Some GPs, however, are uncomfortable with this and look at the UK system and see some advantages:

> We have no electronic clinical records, only very sophisticated billing systems. Management of patients' health is not systematic, and inevit-ably becomes focused upon illness instead of health. There probably is more preventative health activity in Canada because doctors can bill for procedures, but it isn't at all systematic.
>
> UK GPs have incentives to keep their patients healthy because they get paid by capitation, and ironically because they don't have enough time. We are not incentivised to keep patients healthy and it could be argued we have perverse incentives to keep patients ill.
>
> (GP in a hi-tech health centre in a city centre)

Critics of the Canadian system say that it gives doctors incentives to provide many short visits, but no incentives – in fact disincentives – to fix multiple problems in one visit, or to provide education or counselling activities at the same time. Put simply, doctors who choose to have longer visits, and hence treat fewer patients daily, see in effect their remuneration reduced.

Canadian critics of the UK system argue that capitation carries an incentive to under-service because payment is unrelated to the quantity of services provided. Moreover, a system of capitation that requires individuals to enrol with one particular general practitioner or group of healthcare providers reduces a patient's freedom to choose their own healthcare provider.

One of the comments made by a GP in Canada was:

> UK GPs simply don't have enough time to deal with patients. I couldn't possibly deal properly with a patient in only 20 minutes.
>
> (Suburban GP)

Ultimately, most of the arguments come down to money:[66]

> The big difference here compared to many other countries is the remuneration of physicians. To me, this is a great barrier to reforming the system. I personally think that maintaining a fee-for-service form of remuneration is inconsistent with moving to a purchaser–provider model. I do not think that a purchaser–provider model will work with a fee-for-service form of remuneration.
>
> (Professor Cam Donaldson, in evidence
> to the Romanow Commission)

Policy is driven either by cost containment or attempts to modify individual physicians' behaviours by financial incentives, where in all three systems considered the GPs are independent contractors. However, there is a degree of cynicism amongst many about the doctor's attitude to capitation-based remuneration:

> The Ministry sees capitation as a means of cost containment and promoting more health prevention activities. The doctors, and especially the Ontario Medical Association, see capitation as an additional service that can be billed for.
>
> (Healthcare manager)

In the province of Ontario, the chosen vehicle of primary care reform (PCR) has been the primary care network (PCN). In the PCR sites, this network includes physicians at one or more locations who will enrol patients for the provision and coordination of primary care services. In May 1998, the Ministry and the Ontario Medical Association (OMA) jointly announced their proposal for pilot networks.[67]

The Provincial Government set the following goals:

- improved access
- improved quality and continuity of care
- increased patient and provider satisfaction with the healthcare system
- increased cost-effectiveness of healthcare services.

Primary care networks share the following common elements:

- population-based funding for physician services
- enrolment of patients
- improved access
- coordination and continuity of care
- evaluation.

Central to the proposal was the reimbursement mechanism for physicians. All physicians participating in the reform were to be compensated based upon one of two population-based payment arrangements. The funding began to introduce needs-based payments through modification of rates based on age and sex and other variables as they learned more and refined the method of compensation. It was also intended to provide incentives to encourage more physicians to work as part of a team with other physicians and with other primary care providers.

Patients were required to enrol with one primary care physician in a PCN at a time; enrolment imparts a commitment between the patient and the physician in the PCN for the management and acceptance of primary healthcare within the network.

The PCNs were also the vehicle for introducing a range of other reforms, including greater opportunities for nurse practitioners and the greater use of IT and telephone triage systems.

The first evaluation report was published in 2001 on behalf of the Provincial Government.[68] The key findings were:

- The evaluation covered 11 active PCNs: eight PCNs in Hamilton and one each in Chatham, Paris and Kingston. In all networks there appears to be greater interaction among healthcare providers than prior to PCR.
- Generally individuals described the contract negotiation process as long and arduous, and that it took up far more time in meetings than was anticipated. The contract negotiation process was difficult for every network; however, physicians were generally satisfied with their contract except for those under the reformed fee-for-service payment model.
- The plan for the primary care pilot included seven sites: Hamilton, Kingston, Chatham, Paris, Parry Sound, Ottawa and Thunder Bay. To date four of these sites (Hamilton, Kingston, Chatham and Paris) are active and have established primary care networks. Parry Sound and Ottawa have signed their legal agreements and are in the process of setting up networks.
- Many physicians identified rostering as the biggest challenge to starting up their primary care network. There was general consensus that the enrolment process was tedious and very labour intensive. For many physician offices it required evening and weekend work and impinged on administration and patient care time. Some practices hired extra staff to assist with rostering.
- All of the networks are using the capitation method of physician remuneration, except Chatham which is using the reformed fee-for-service method. Some of the issues raised with respect to the capitation method include roster limits, outside use or negation rates, inclusions and exclusions of services/procedures in the capitation rate, capitation rates for the elderly, capitation rate increases and on-call coverage.

- A much lower level of satisfaction was reported by physicians using the reformed fee-for-service method. Issues include a lower than expected level of income in the initial stages, difficulty accessing the benefits of the bonus codes, rostering requirements and on-call coverage.
- There are currently seven nurse practitioners working in the PCNs.
- The most striking feature of teletriage utilisation to date has been the high volume of calls.
- Between October and December 2000, rostered patients made a total of 4840 calls to the teletriage.
- The IT component of PCR is extremely important to physicians. A cost-sharing arrangement is in place by which the Ministry pays two-thirds of the cost of new IT systems and the physician pays one-third of the cost.
- Despite the many implementation challenges, at this stage in the reform physicians in most networks report a fairly high level of satisfaction with PCR. Most of the physicians interviewed are more satisfied now than they were prior to its implementation.
- Physicians in the Chatham PCN report a very low level of satisfaction with PCR.
- Based on patient focus groups at two of the PCN sites, there was general agreement that the quality of care received by patients was directly related to the way the individual doctor chooses to approach their profession. Former patients enrolled in a Health Service Organization (HSO) noticed little change under primary care reform.

Viewed from the UK, the first observation is that the rate and scope of change is small, covering 220 000 patients in total with 145 physicians, or just under 2% of the provincial population. This may not be a bad thing. Whilst the practice nurse innovations are seen as a success, seven practice nurses is not a huge innovation amongst 145 physicians.

The biggest discriminator amongst physicians is the payment mode. The satisfaction with capitation when compared with the reformed fee-for-service method suggests that capitation fee levels may not be sustainable in a wider implementation. The report is noticeably reticent on claims over cost-effectiveness in spite of it being one of the four core goals:

> The doctors will go for capitation provided that it doesn't reduce their overall income. This is incompatible with the province making overall cost savings.
>
> (Healthcare manager)

The PCNs have now evolved into the Ontario Family Health Networks (OFHNs). These are still evolving and the interested reader is referred to the OFHN website for more information.[69]

Whilst primary care reform is a major theme of the Romanow Commission's final report, apart from some proposals on diverting finance from secondary to primary care, the report is noticeably vaguer in this area than others on how its noble ideals are to be realised.

## The problems of rural populations

Canada shares with Australia a large land mass with its population concentrated in a small area, with all the major urban centres close to the country's southern boundary. The total population of Canada was 31 414 000[5] in July 2002, or approximately 50% more than Australia and just over half that of the UK.

The percentage of the population living in rural areas in the 2001 census is shown in Table 8.1.[5]

**Table 8.1**   Percentage of population living in rural areas (2001 census)

| Province | % Rural | Number |
|---|---|---|
| CANADA | 20 | 6 098 883 |
| Ontario | 15 | 1 747 499 |
| Quebec | 20 | 1 420 330 |
| British Columbia | 15 | 597 885 |
| Alberta | 19 | 569 647 |
| Nova Scotia | 44 | 400 998 |
| New Brunswick | 50 | 361 596 |
| Saskatchewan | 36 | 349 897 |
| Manitoba | 28 | 314 262 |
| Newfoundland | 42 | 216 734 |
| Prince Edward Island | 55 | 74 619 |
| Nunavut | 68 | 18 056 |
| Northwest Territories | 42 | 15 529 |
| Yukon | 41 | 11 831 |

These figures need a little bit of care in interpretation. By UK standards the territories of Nunavut, Northwest Territories and Yukon are very rural, and even the Atlantic provinces are more like the Highlands of Scotland than the Sussex Downs! Data from Statistics Canada and CIHI, cited by the Romanow report,[60] demonstrates the poorer outcomes for rural populations:

- Life expectancy for people in predominantly rural regions is less than the Canadian average.
- Disability rates are higher in smaller communities.
- Rates for accidents, poisoning and violence are also higher in smaller communities.
- People living in remote northern communities are the least healthy and have the lowest life and disability-free life expectancies.

In its 2002 report, Statistics Canada identifies ten different peer groups and compares health outcomes (*see* Table 8.2).[5]

Group C from the northern rural areas consistently performs worse than other groups, including the rural populations from the prairies, in terms of health outcomes and health behaviours, although in terms of psychosocial factors, other peer groups are worse (*see* Figure 8.1a, b and c).

**Table 8.2**  Comparison of ten different peer groups and health outcomes[5]

| Group | Regions | % Pop. | Characteristics |
|---|---|---|---|
| A | 5 | 17.4 | Metropolitan areas such as Toronto, Montréal and Vancouver<br>• Average population size over one million<br>• High percentage (32.0%) of visible minority population<br>• Low percentage (0.6%) of aboriginal population<br>• High average number of years of schooling (13.9 years)<br>• High inequality of income distribution (median share = 18.8%) |
| B | 8 | 16.5 | Large urban centres with a relatively high population density<br>• Average population size over 500 000<br>• High percentage (20.2%) of visible minority population<br>• Low percentage (1.5%) of aboriginal population<br>• High average number of years of schooling (13.9 years) |
| C | 6 | 0.4 | Mostly northern health regions<br>• High percentage (75.5%) of aboriginal population<br>• High unemployment rate (17.2%)<br>• Low density of population (3.9 people per square kilometre)<br>• Low percentage (0.9%) of visible minority population<br>• Low average number of years of schooling (10.6 years) |
| D | 9 | 2.6 | Mostly eastern health regions<br>• High unemployment rate (27.7%)<br>• Low percentage (0.5%) of visible minority population<br>• Low percentage (9.1%) of inter-municipality migrants<br>• Low average personal income (slightly over $18 000) |
| E | 13 | 2.8 | Mostly rural health regions in the prairies<br>• High percentage (16.5%) of people aged 65 or older<br>• Low percentage (1.1%) of visible minority population<br>• Low average personal income (slightly over $20 000) |
| F | 13 | 2.2 | Mostly northern health regions<br>• High percentage (17.2%) of aboriginal population<br>• Low density of population (0.5 people per square kilometre)<br>• Low inequality of income distribution (median share = 23.6%)<br>• High percentage (22.8%) of inter-municipality migrants |
| G | 21 | 5.5 | Mostly rural health regions in the prairies<br>• Low unemployment rate (7.1%)<br>• Low percentage (10.4%) of lone-parent families<br>• Low percentage (13.8%) of people with low income |

*Continued*

**Table 8.2**  Continued

| Group | Regions | % Pop. | Characteristics |
|---|---|---|---|
| H | 22 | 23.2 | Health regions mostly in Québec and its neighbouring provinces<br>• Low population growth (0.6%)<br>• High to moderate unemployment rate (11.2%)<br>• Moderate percentage (14.9%) of lone-parent families |
| I | 34 | 23.5 | Health regions mostly in Ontario<br>• High percentage (85.9%) of residents commuting to the nearby urban centres<br>• Moderate to high percentage (13.5%) of people aged 65 or over |
| J | 8 | 5.9 | Mostly sub-metropolitan health regions<br>• High population growth (4.3%)<br>• Low unemployment rate (7.5%)<br>• High percentage (24.0%) of inter-municipality migrants<br>• Low percentage (13.9%) of children living in low-income households<br>• Low inequality of income distribution (median share = 24.4%)<br>• High average number of years of schooling (13.5 years) |

Health Canada established the Office of Rural Health in 1998 to deal with the health issues of rural Canadians. Interestingly, their figures differ from those of the official Government census, claiming up to nine million Canadians live in rural areas. This has been recognised and a policy paper was produced in 2002 on a common definition.[70]

Telehealth has been used less in Canada than Australia. It was a major theme of the Health Transition Fund (HTF) project:[71]

> The telehealth-related projects all saw telehealth as a way to improve rural health services delivery. For instance, the demonstration project *Telemedicine Serving Québec Regions: a demonstration project* in the Magdalen Islands (QC425) was intended to bring diagnostic, treatment and rehabilitation services to rural and remote areas; to reduce the number of patient transfers to urban centres and to provide continuing education to healthcare practitioners on the Magdalen Islands.
>
> The *First Nations National Telehealth Research Project* (NA402) had similar objectives. It pointed out that since over a third of First Nations and Inuit communities were found in remote or isolated locations, telehealth had the potential to even out geographic disparities in access to healthcare. Other projects (e.g. NA403, QC323) hoped that telehealth would lower the costs associated with travel to distant medical facilities or make continuing education programs accessible to rural practitioners.

(a)

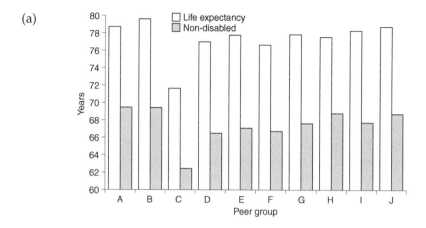

(b)

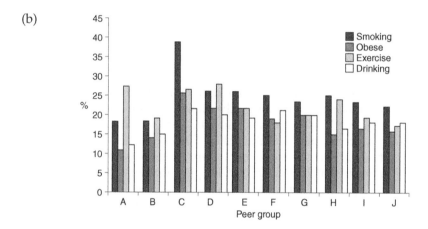

(c)

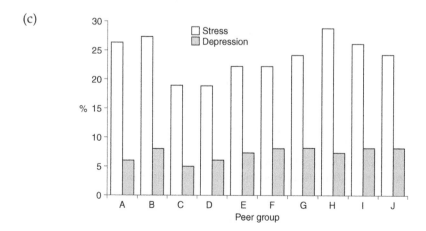

**Figure 8.1**   (a) Life expectancy and non-disabled life expectancies for the different groups; (b) Negative health behaviours for the different groups; (c) Psycho-social factors for the different groups.

One project had a more ambitious goal: Québec's Hôpital Sainte-Justine telehealth project, *Supraregional Mother–Child Network* (QC305), planned to establish the réseau mère–enfant (mother–child network) among the hospitals in Montréal and the surrounding rural regions, with a view to improving access to, and the quality of, care for mothers and their infants by coordinating the work of the participating hospitals by means of telehealth.

It should be noted that the use of telehealth has expanded substantially in recent years. Previously, it was used primarily by physicians for diagnosis, consultation and the transfer of medical data such as X-ray images, as well as for delivering continuing medical education programs at a distance. More recently, as exemplified by some of the HTF projects, the field of telehealth has become considerably broader, comprising tele-triage, tele-monitoring (e.g. NA161, NA403), tele-home care (e.g. ON121) and tele-rehabilitation.

Most of the telehealth-related HTF projects reported user satisfaction. As an example, the *Telecentres for Education and Community Health (TEACH) Project* (NA366) reported that 90 per cent of its clients rated the telehealth facilities as good or excellent and that almost all of its clients would use telehealth services again.

Several projects had successfully used telehealth for patient education (e.g. NA403) and to bring continuing education programs to rural-based practitioners (e.g. NA402, QC323). The latter was considered very important from a practitioner recruitment and retention perspective because it might help reduce the sense of professional isolation or practitioners' concern that they were not keeping up with developments in their disciplines. Telehealth helped to reduce the number of patient transfers and patients' need to travel long distances in order to seek medical care. The TEACH project (NA366) reported that some patients who had consulted specialists by means of telehealth saved as much as $3000 in travel costs. According to the *Nephrology Telemedicine Project* (NA403), 55 per cent of the patients involved in the project believed that the program had reduced their travel costs and had cut down significantly the amount of time they had to spend travelling to hospitals for dialysis treatments. The results reported above, though generally favourable, were often achieved at substantial costs. Although the evaluation studies were not designed to be a cost–benefit analysis, some reports did raise concerns about the costs involved and wondered if they were justified. For example, the *First Nations National Telehealth Research Project* (NA402) was an expensive initiative, with infrastructure costs averaging $245 000 to $305 000 per site.

At the same time, utilization in some of the telehealth projects was very low. For instance, although Alberta's *Keeweetinok Lakes Regional Health Authority Telehealth Project* (AB301-19) was put in place at a cost of $3.5 million, the project evaluator concluded that there were insufficient telehealth interaction episodes to indicate whether or not telehealth was effective.

Similarly, as pointed out by the evaluator of the *Nephrology Telemedicine Project* (NA403) in New Brunswick, although expensive telehealth paraphernalia, such as electrocardiogram equipment, tele-radiology systems and computers, had been purchased, they were never or seldom used during the project.

However, it is worth pointing out that telehealth programs typically entail a substantial front-end investment in technology and infrastructure installation. As well, since many rural and remote communities do not have a large population, the potential telehealth clientele is small. Thus, the initial cost per telehealth contact episode tends to be very high. As the utilization rate increases or as technology becomes more affordable, the per contact episode cost is likely to decline.

In spite of a degree of enthusiasm and a number of successful pilot projects, telehealth does not appear to be having the impact that it has in parts of Queensland and the Northern Territories. Whilst cost is a factor in Canada, it is also a factor in Australia.

One reason suggested in Australia for the impact that telehealth had had there was the tradition of remote services, such as the Royal Flying Doctor Service, which had prepared the general population for such services. There is no such tradition in Canada.

In Canada, a higher priority has been placed upon incentives to recruit and retain healthcare professionals in rural areas.

One person recounted how her community had problems recruiting a doctor:

> We couldn't get a doctor to come to our town. No one was prepared to come with the implications for their personal remuneration. So the town got together to build a new health centre, to attract a doctor.
> The initiative was successful and the efforts of the community were sufficient to convince a doctor to come. In other areas, coverage is effectively provided by a nurse practitioner with the support of a doctor somewhere at a considerable distance.
> (Ex-hospital CEO, now living in a rural community)

One of the most effective uses of telehealth technology may be to support isolated healthcare professionals by offering specialist advice and support for GPs and nurse practitioners, as well as simple human contact.

It was suggested by one of my interviewees that there was scope for a scheme for encouraging new young doctors to gain experience in rural contexts:

> It's sometimes difficult for new young doctors to find employment. They could be offered jobs with incentives to move to rural areas.
> (Health manager)

One possible model would be the Australian HECS reimbursement scheme allowing doctors to work off their debts from study in posts in rural areas. However, the Romanow report warns against simplistic solutions:[60]

> The problems with the supply of physicians in rural and remote communities demand solutions. But the experiences of many provinces and territories as well as OECD countries suggest that short-term solutions

aimed at increasing the overall supply of physicians do not necessarily translate into improvements in their supply in these communities. Provincial and territorial governments have tried providing incentives to encourage physicians to move to rural areas through higher pay or other financial incentives. In other cases, governments have tried to limit where new physicians can practice in order to encourage more of them to work in rural communities.

Physicians typically object to measures that limit their ability to choose where they practice. Part of the answer certainly lies in increasing physicians' exposure to rural settings as part of their education and training. With increased exposure to, and experience in, rural settings, the likelihood of graduating doctors wanting to practice in rural settings increases (BCMA 2002). Recent efforts by the Society of Rural Physicians of Canada and the College of Family Physicians of Canada to develop national curricula and guidelines are a step in the right direction. But there is much more to be done.

(p.163)

# Conclusions

## Are the policy values carried into practice?

The Canadian system prides itself on being a public system. This is hard to defend without qualification. The system is delivered largely by private organisations. The percentage of expenditure derived from the public sector is considerably less than the UK and comparable with Australia which is effectively a publicly regulated private system.

On the other hand, the Canadian system does deliver to most Canadians a package of medical services free at the point of delivery which is the envy of the world. Waiting times, whilst sometimes causing concern, are in order of magnitude better than in the UK. In the words of one interviewee:

> UK waiting times would bring down provincial Governments in Canada.
> (Health manager)

or the response from a member of the audience after a presentation about fundholding on a previous visit to Canada in 1998:

> That's a load of c**p! Its impossible that a Government that spends so little on healthcare would want to introduce a cost control mechanism.
> (Doctor)

The Canada Health Act remains dominant in its influence. The use of the phrase 'medically necessary' has skewed developments along a medically dominated course, and reinforced the power of the doctors and the medical associations. This has put a brake upon reforms, which whilst primarily aimed at cost containment, have the potential to improve health in areas such as systematic surveillance.

At the same time, it does seem anomalous that drugs prescribed outside hospital, which surely meet the criteria of 'medically necessary' but are not a 'service', are not covered by the Act.

The issue of cost remains a challenge for any public system. However:

- Canada provides some of the best evidence of the cost-effectiveness of public healthcare compared to private provision.
- The USA, which is an obvious comparator, spends far more and achieves less in terms of population coverage and health outcomes.
- Australia spends less but has worse health outcomes.
- The UK spends a lot less but has waiting times that are undreamed of in Canada, and is increasing spending dramatically at present.

The problems in rural areas do seem to challenge the principle of universality. How can the same service be provided in Nunavut as in central Toronto? On the other hand, there is no evidence from Australia that a private system provides a better or more universal service.

Finally, it is impossible for outsiders to underestimate the importance of the Provincial/Federal Government relationship in the Canadian system. It is likely to be this relationship which will determine if the Canada Health Act survives. The Romanow report,[60] recently published, recognises many of the issues raised and largely reaffirms the emphases of the Canada Health Act. It does, however, call for a significant increase in investment and for some measures that will be unpopular in some provinces. It remains to be seen if this new vision of Canadian healthcare will be put into practice.

# Strengths, weaknesses, opportunities and threats in healthcare in Canada

The study has revealed the following SWOTs (*see* Box 8.2).

---

**Box 8.2**  SWOTs in healthcare in Canada

| *Strengths* | *Weaknesses* |
|---|---|
| • Universality | • Medical focus |
| • Health outcomes | • Exceptions to coverage, notably drugs |
| • Value for money, cf. the USA | • Recruitment and retention in rural areas |
| | • Limited services in rural areas |

| *Opportunities* | *Threats* |
|---|---|
| • Primary care reform | • Provincial/Federal relationship |
| • Romanow Commission | • Diversity between provinces |
| | • Cost control |
| | • Resistance to change from clinicians |

The biggest threats to the Canadian system are Professor Bob Evans' 'zombies':[12] the problems with controlling demand in a public system may lead people to embrace more private provision. There is little evidence from Australia (and less from the USA) that this will lead to cost containment.

The second threat remains the comfort of the physicians with the current situation. They enjoy a position of enviable financial advantage, considerable power and status. They have little incentive to engage in reform which would dilute this. The danger, if they do not, is that they may simply bring the whole edifice crashing down around them.

# CHAPTER 9

# Driver 1: finance

## Financing health: an overview

The first driver we shall consider is finance. Finance drives health policy in two ways:

- How much money does a country believe that it should spend upon healthcare?
- How should that money be found?

The traditional measure of healthcare expenditure is % Gross Domestic Product. In other words, this is the proportion of available national income spent on health care.

The UK traditionally is shown to spend less of its income on healthcare than most comparable countries (*see* Figure 9.1).

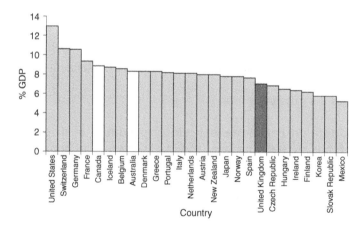

**Figure 9.1**  National expenditure on healthcare expressed as % GDP.[72]

As noted in Chapter 4, this expenditure has risen consistently up to the early 1990s, when it has generally plateaued or reduced. In the early 1990s, in a number of countries expenditure approached or exceeded 10% of GDP. This appears to have been an unacceptable level in all countries except the USA, leading to health-care reform aimed at cost control (*see* Table 9.1).

The impact of cost-containment reform is shown by the fact that in 12 of the 15 highest spenders, expenditure is declining as a percentage of national income by 2000. These cost-containment reforms have been the principal driver in healthcare during the past ten years.

**Table 9.1** High spenders in healthcare 1990–2000*

|  | 1990 | 1991 | 1992 | 1993 | 1994 | 1995 | 1996 | 1997 | 1998 | 1999 | 2000 |
|---|---|---|---|---|---|---|---|---|---|---|---|
| United States | 11.9 | 12.6 | 13 | 13.3 | 13.2 | **13.3** | 13.2 | 13 | 12.9 | 13 | 13 |
| Switzerland | 8.5 | 9.2 | 9.6 | 9.6 | 9.8 | 10 | 10.4 | 10.4 | 10.6 | 10.7 | **10.7** |
| Germany | 8.7 |  | 9.9 | 9.9 | 10.2 | 10.6 | **10.9** | 10.7 | 10.6 | 10.7 | 10.6 |
| France | 8.6 | 8.9 | 9.1 | 9.5 | 9.4 | **9.6** | **9.6** | 9.4 | 9.3 | 9.4 | 9.5 |
| Canada | 9 | 9.7 | **10** | 9.8 | 9.5 | 9.1 | 8.9 | 8.9 | 9.1 | 9.2 | 9.1 |
| Iceland | 7.9 | 8.1 | 8.1 | **8.3** | 8 | 8.2 | 8.2 | 8 | 8.3 | 8.7 | **8.9** |
| Belgium | 7.4 | 7.7 | 7.9 | 8.1 | 7.9 | 8.7 | **8.8** | 8.5 | 8.5 | 8.7 | 8.7 |
| Australia | 7.8 | 8 | 8.1 | 8.1 | 8.1 | 8.2 | 8.3 | 8.4 | **8.5** | 8.4 | 8.3 |
| Denmark | 8.5 | 8.4 | 8.5 | **8.8** | 8.5 | 8.2 | 8.3 | 8.2 | 8.4 | 8.5 | 8.3 |
| Greece | 7.5 | 7.8 | 7.2 | 8.1 | **8.9** | **8.9** | **8.9** | 8.7 | 8.7 | 8.7 | 8.3 |
| Portugal | 6.2 | 6.8 | 7 | 7.3 | 7.3 | 8.3 | 8.5 | **8.6** | 8.3 | 8.4 | 8.2 |
| Italy | 8 | 8.3 | **8.4** | 8.1 | 7.8 | 7.4 | 7.5 | 7.7 | 7.7 | 7.8 | 8.1 |
| Netherlands | 8 | 8.2 | 8.4 | **8.5** | 8.4 | 8.4 | 8.3 | 8.2 | 8.1 | 8.2 | 8.1 |
| Austria | 7.1 | 7.1 | 7.5 | 7.9 | 7.9 | 8.6 | **8.7** | 8 | 8 | 8.1 | 8 |
| New Zealand | 6.9 | 7.4 | **7.5** | 7.2 | 7.2 | 7.2 | 7.2 | 7.5 | 7.9 | 7.9 | **8** |

*High spenders are those spending 8% or more of GDP on healthcare in 2000. The peak expenditure is highlighted in bold.

The second financial driver is how the money is to be provided. This is generally characterised as being either:

- public – raised from general taxation, or
- private – paid directly by the patient, often through a private insurance scheme.

The OECD defines the difference thus:[73]

- Public expenditure on healthcare is health expenditure incurred by public funds. Public funds are state, regional and local Government bodies and social security schemes. Public capital formation on health includes publicly financed investment in health facilities plus capital transfers to the private sector for hospital construction and equipment.
- Private expenditure on healthcare is the privately funded part of total health expenditure. Private sources of funds include out-of-pocket payments (both over-the-counter and cost-sharing), private insurance programmes, charities and occupational healthcare.

In Australia, Canada and the United Kingdom, public funding is largely derived from general tax revenue, while in other European systems, such as Germany and the Netherlands, most of the public funds allocated to healthcare are raised by the social insurance system through employers' and employees' contributions.

Canadians generally regard themselves as having a public system. The OECD data[73] on the percentage of healthcare expenditure provided by public funding show that the perceptions of respondents in the interviews are not reflected in reality. The Australian system was characterised as a predominantly private system. The Canadian system was characterised as a public system. The UK system was characterised as a public system with a small but significant private sector.

In reality, all healthcare systems are hybrids: they have a combination of public and private involvement in financing and delivering healthcare. The characteristics of each healthcare system also vary from country to country depending on their political economy and structure of government, as well as on the values of their respective society.

OECD data,[73] illustrated in Figure 9.2, show that the UK has the greatest percentage of expenditure from the public purse and that the Australian system has recently risen sharply, and actually overtaken the Canadian percentage in recent years. In general there has been a decline in the percentage of public health expenditure over the decade in Canada. In Australia, the public percentage of expenditure has risen steadily since the mid 1990s. This is at a time when the Government is promoting private healthcare insurance to a very great extent.

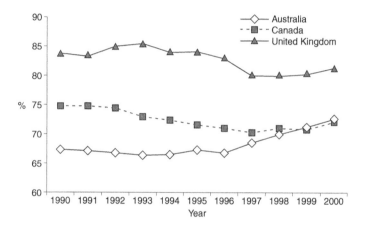

**Figure 9.2** Percentage of healthcare expenditure funded from public expenditure.[73]

# How finance has driven policy in the UK

The UK has traditionally spent less on healthcare than almost any other major developed country, with the possible exception of Ireland. This has produced an efficient system but one which has major problems with access to healthcare, which have been highlighted previously.

*The NHS Plan*,[74] which outlines Government policy for the NHS, details four alternative mechanisms for the future of funding:

> **3.3** Essentially those who argue that the NHS is not sustainable advocate making one – or a combination – of four reforms:
>
> - *private insurance*: the Government should provide incentives to people to help them make their own arrangements and payments for healthcare in an attempt to ease pressure on the NHS and to seek to raise the total national expenditure on health;

- *charges*: the Government should introduce new charges for services as an attempt to encourage people to use the health service more responsibly and raise more revenue for the NHS;
- *social insurance*: the Government should move wholesale to a French- or German-style system for funding healthcare where funds are raised predominantly from employees and employers rather than from the population as a whole;
- *rationing the service down to a fixed core*: the Government should ration services to a limited list of procedures as a response to medical advances.

**3.4** Each of these proposals has been examined against two key criteria which should underpin any modern healthcare funding system:

- *efficiency*: testing whether or not the proposal would achieve its proposed end and whether or not it provides the greatest possible health improvement and healthcare within the funding available;
- *equity*: analysing how well the proposal would match financial contributions to ability to pay, and how well it would match healthcare to health needs.

### Private health insurance
**3.5** When people propose the Government should boost national spending on health, by providing incentives to individuals to make provision for their own healthcare needs, they normally mean tax incentives for individuals and/or employers for making contributions towards private medical insurance.

### The efficiency test
**3.6** This approach is inefficient in five respects:

**3.7** First, as a policy its effects are likely to be minimal without a strong element of compulsion. In 1990 the previous Government introduced tax relief on private medical insurance for the over-60s. Despite annual public spending of £140 million on these incentives, the numbers of subscribers to private medical insurance rose by only about 50 000 in seven years. This 1.6% increase therefore had only a marginal effect on the NHS. More recent experience from Australia confirms this analysis. Three years of experimenting with increasingly costly public subsidies – totalling £1 billion – appears to have merely stopped a long-term decline in the coverage of private health insurance. These subsidies have mainly benefited those already with insurance and so far may have added much more to public spending than to private funding.

**3.8** Second, using public money to pay for tax incentives diverts funds from the public healthcare system. The cost of providing tax relief to those who already have private health insurance would be significantly over £500 million – the so-called dead-weight cost. Unless taxes were to rise or spending in another area of government were to fall, that would mean the NHS budget being reduced by the same amount.

**3.9** Third, it is misleading to presume that incentives for people to 'go private' saves the public sector money. This is because the saving to the

NHS is likely to be outweighed by the dead-weight costs of subsidising those who already have private medical insurance. A recent report from the Institute for Fiscal Studies concluded that 'it is extremely unlikely that the cost of any such subsidy to private medical insurance would be less than the NHS expenditure saved'. In other words, switching public funding from NHS expenditure to spending on tax relief could reduce health spending overall.

**3.10** Fourth, the development of genetic testing will affect the coverage and cost of voluntary private health insurance. Healthcare risks will become more transparent. As a result, premiums will rise to reflect high-risk subscribers' potential claims, reducing the affordability of cover, and lower risk subscribers will drop out. The combined effect will be to erode the risk pool on which private health insurance depends.

**3.11** Fifth, whether or not the introduction of tax relief increased the overall volume of healthcare, it would certainly inflate its costs:

- *labour costs*: currently there is no surplus of doctors and nurses in our country. The previous Government considered the introduction of tax relief in 1988. As Nigel Lawson, the then Chancellor of the Exchequer, concluded: 'If we simply boost demand, for example by tax concessions to the private sector, without improving supply, the result would not be so much a growth in private healthcare, but higher prices;
- *fragmentation*: the more fragmented commissioning of healthcare becomes, the more prices would be likely to rise. In the USA, for example, pharmaceutical prices are on average 75% higher than in Britain. This is at least in part due to the fragmentation of healthcare purchasing;
- *administration*: administrative costs would rise significantly. The costs of management and administration are much higher under private insurance because of the bureaucracy needed to assess risk, set premiums, design complex benefit schedules and review, pay or refuse claims. These raised costs impact on hospital budgets. Administrative costs in America are up to 15% higher than in Canada, largely because of the cost of insurance processing. The implication is that much of any increase in private medical insurance in Britain would go in administrative costs, with no direct benefits to patients.

**The equity test**

**3.12** Private medical insurance is inequitable. Subsidising private health insurance will use taxpayers funds to expand two-tier access to healthcare, reducing equitable access to needed care. The costs of private health insurance per individual are substantial. For a 65-year-old, private health insurance costs around 50% more than the equivalent NHS cost.

**3.13** Private medical insurance shifts the burden of paying for healthcare from the healthy, young and wealthy to the unhealthy, old and poor. The cost of private health insurance rises, the older and sicker the person is. Indeed, beyond a certain age, and with chronic conditions, it is virtually impossible to get private insurance cover. Tax relief for private health insurance by definition is regressive. It offers public subsidies to the better off and is meaningless for the worst off.

**3.14** This view is borne out by findings from a large-scale research study in the early 1990s which looked at the costs across income classes of healthcare in Europe and America. It concluded: 'The two countries with predominately private financing systems – Switzerland and the US – have the most regressive structures overall.... The group of countries with the next most regressive systems are the countries operating the so-called social insurance model, ... countries which rely ... mainly on tax finance ... have the least regressive financing systems.'

### Charges

**3.15** Proponents of patient charges argue that new charges should be introduced for a range of health services to encourage responsible use of resources and raise more revenue for the NHS.

### The efficiency test

**3.16** Where charges are high they generally reduce service use across the board. The most thorough study of charges and cost sharing, the RAND Health Insurance Experiment – a randomised trial undertaken in the USA in the 1970s – found that charges led to less use of preventative care. The available evidence suggests that they are also likely to discourage use of necessary services. As the World Health Organization has recently noted: 'The use of co-payments has the effect of rationing the use of a specific intervention but does not have the effect of rationalising its demand by consumers.' Lower use and delayed access to healthcare services, especially preventive services, may divert demand to more costly parts of the system and may result in higher healthcare costs in the longer term.

**3.17** It is sometimes suggested that these undesirable behavioural effects can be avoided by setting new user charges at a low level. Where charges are low they raise very little cash, which may be off-set by administrative and collection costs. For example, in 1992 New Zealand introduced charges for the use of hospital beds. The difficulty of collecting the charges from patients led to their rapid abolition in 1993 after only a year. Equally, in countries such as France that make widespread use of charges, many individuals take out supplementary insurance just to pay them, thus defeating the object of introducing the charges at all.

### The equity test

**3.18** Charges are inequitable in two important respects. First, new charges increase the proportion of funding from the unhealthy, old and poor compared with the healthy, young and wealthy. In particular, high charges risk worsening access to healthcare by the poor. As the World Heath Organization report – which assessed the United Kingdom as having one of the fairest systems in the world for funding healthcare – concludes: 'Fairness of financial risk protection requires the highest possible degree of separation between contributions and utilisation.'

**3.19** Second, exempting low-income families from user charges can create inequities for those just above the threshold. High user charges with exemptions can create disincentives to earning and working through the imposition of high marginal tax rates.

**3.20** Some European countries do make more use of user charges than Britain. For example, in parts of Sweden in 1996 there were charges for seeing a GP of about £10 per visit and for seeing a consultant of about £20 per consultant. They are able to do so in large part because they tend to compensate people indirectly through the social security benefit system. Even so, in Sweden there is evidence that user charges for visiting primary care doctors have discouraged people from seeking treatment.

### Continental social insurance

**3.21** There are those who advocate maintaining the current role of public funding but shifting wholesale to a social insurance-based model. This is similar to both the German and French healthcare systems. The proponents of this model argue that it leads to larger shares of national income going to healthcare.

### The efficiency test

**3.22** Social insurance systems involve payments from individuals just like tax-financed systems. In the French and German social insurance systems, costs fall predominantly on the employer and employee and so fewer people contribute. An outline estimate from 1997 is that a wholesale switch to funding the NHS predominantly from national insurance contributions would cost an extra £1000 per employee per year using the French model of public healthcare funding and about £700 per employee per year using the German model, without any increase in the total amount of resources going to the NHS. These calculations adjust for the different levels of expenditure in the three countries, i.e. French and German expenditures are assumed to be reduced to current British levels. At 2003–04 levels of funding, additional costs would be the equivalent of £1500 per worker per year using the French model and £1000 using the German model, again, with no addition to currently planned NHS funding.

**3.23** Continental social insurance models are less efficient in several respects.

**3.24** First, because of the design of the social insurance systems in continental Europe, it is not clear that all of the extra spending is spent efficiently. Cost control under European social insurance systems has been weak because payers have acted as financial intermediaries within the healthcare system but have not played a role in scrutinising the performance, efficiency and effectiveness of the system itself. In the words of the German Head of the Federal Association of General Sick Funds: 'Germany pays for a luxury car but gets a medium-range car in return' and 'If we don't look out, our medium-range car will soon be without brakes and wheels.'

**3.25** The French system, despite patient choice, is wasteful in the use of many of its resources. Over-prescribing is common. At only 3%, generic prescribing rates are far lower than the 60% found in Britain. To tackle these inefficiencies France and Germany are turning to healthcare management mechanisms which have been in operation in Britain for many years, such as a GP referral-based system of primary care.

**3.26** Second, in recent years fiscal policy and competitiveness considerations have forced all governments to subject social insurance systems to increasingly tight regulation. By placing caps on contribution rates or expenditure, the national governments in Germany and France now effectively determine overall expenditure under their social insurance systems rather than the social insurance partners. In other words, levels of health funding are increasingly unrelated to the system of raising finance and increasingly related to how much the economy can afford and the level of priority placed on health spending by the public.

**The equity test**
**3.27** The extent to which social insurance is equitable depends upon the form of the particular scheme.

**Rationing to a core service**
**3.28** The fourth solution sometimes suggested is that the NHS should be restricted or 'rationed' to a defined core of individual conditions or treatments. There are several problems with this suggestion.

**3.29** First, advocates of this position usually have great difficulty specifying what they would rule out. The sort of treatments that commonly feature include varicose veins, wisdom teeth extraction or cosmetic procedures. The problem is that these sort of services account for less than 0.5% of the NHS budget, and are not major cost-drivers for the future. Instead, the vast majority of spending – and spending increases – go on childbirth, elderly care and major conditions such as cancer, heart disease and mental health problems.

**3.30** The second major problem is that different patients under different circumstances often derive differing benefits from the same treatment.

**3.31** The NHS is not a system under which each patient only gets a fixed 'ration' of healthcare, regardless of their personal need and circumstances. The fact that a patient has previously been treated for one condition will not of itself prevent her or him from being treated for subsequent conditions. If, however, 'rationing' merely means that it has never and will never be possible in practice to provide all the healthcare theoretically possible, then it is true of every healthcare system in the world.

*The NHS Plan* concludes that the NHS funding mechanism will not be radically reformed, but changed from within by increasing accountability, efficiency and prioritisation:[74]

> **3.32** The issue is not whether the NHS – just like every other public or private health service – has to set priorities and make choices. The issue is how those choices are made. Under the NHS, treatment is based on peoples' ability to benefit. We are in a period of significant expansion

of health service resources. The issue is how to improve decisions about how those expanded resources are used. We can no longer leave to chance decisions about how treatment is provided, how demand is managed and how costs are driven. National Service Frameworks and the broad priorities set out in this *NHS Plan* provide the context. The National Institute for Clinical Excellence, supported by its new Citizens Council (see paragraph 10.20), will help the NHS to focus its growing resources on those interventions and treatments that will best improve peoples' health. By pointing out which treatments are less clinically cost-effective, it will help free up financial headroom for faster uptake of more appropriate and clinically cost-effective interventions. This is the right way to set priorities: not a crudely rationed core service.

# The private sector in the UK NHS

In reality, there is a significant increased use of the private sector and private finance. However, it is on the supply side rather than the consumer side.

The proportion of people who purchase private healthcare insurance in the United Kingdom has historically been low, but has steadily grown in recent years to 11.5% of the population. Examination of the socio-economic status of people with private insurance indicates that it is heavily skewed towards higher socio-economic groups. The percentage of people with private insurance varies considerably across the country, approaching 20% in London, whereas in Scotland it is as low as 5%.

The Government is not seeking, in contrast to Australia, to expand the use of private healthcare. Instead it is using its Private Finance Initiative (PFI) to rapidly expand capital investment to increase and modernise capacity.

The PFI is a controversial way of procuring large capital projects that were previously funded by public expenditure and included in the Government's borrowing requirements. The scheme was introduced in 1992 by the Conservative Government but was enthusiastically adopted and extended by the Labour administration in 1997.[75]

Under the PFI a hospital has to be designed, built, financed and operated by a private sector consortium for a period of up to 60 years, but more typically 25 to 30 years. The private consortium will be regularly paid from public money depending on its performance throughout that period. At the end of the period, control of the project can switch to the public sector. If the consortium misses performance targets, it will be paid less.

The attraction of the PFI for the Government is that it avoids making expensive one-off payments to build large-scale projects. By transferring risk to the private sector the PFI also gets round tough public rules that prevent public bodies raising private cash. The attraction for private companies is that if the project is delivered as specified, the PFI guarantees regular payments for an extended period.

Critics of such schemes have criticised them as a 'build now, pay more later' system that also involves paying large sums to consultants to set up complex contracts. As with any form of hire purchase, buying a product over a long period of time is more expensive than buying with cash up front. Critics point out that governments can borrow cash at a cheaper rate than the private sector.

What particularly frustrates opponents of the PFI is that in many parts of Europe public bodies can raise private cash under more relaxed borrowing rules known as the General Government Financial Deficit (GGFD).

The Government claims that the PFI is a way of providing immediate improvements to Britain's crumbling infrastructure and introduces private sector efficiencies to public services. But in the first wave of PFI projects, those same efficiencies were seen as corner cutting. The first PFI hospitals contained 30% fewer beds than those planned under traditional procurement methods. The buildings were dismissed as being poorly designed by the Government's own advisors.

There is some evidence that the more recent PFI projects are delivering greater value for money as the public sector gains more experience of the initiative. Greater confidence from banks has also led to cheaper borrowing for the projects. But it will take a further 20 to 25 years when the first contracts have been completed before the real cost of the PFI can be judged.

The PFI remains a crucial mechanism for the UK Government in its attempts to improve the NHS:[76]

> **4.8** The Private Finance Initiative (PFI) continues to help us deliver the largest hospital building programme in the history of the NHS. On current plans, PFI will provide nearly £800 million capital for 2002–03. This represents 28.4 per cent of total NHS capital spending in this year.
>
> A further eight of the 'first wave' of major PFI schemes finish construction and become operational (Greenwich, Calderdale, North Durham, South Manchester, Norfolk & Norwich, Hereford, Barnet & Chase Farm and Worcestershire), making a total of 11 in the past two years. Two more are expected to be completed by the end of 2002.
>
> In February 2001 a further 29 new hospitals, each with a capital value of over £20 million, were given the go-ahead under the PFI procurement procedure. Several of these are timetabled to go out to tender during 2002.
>
> As well as the programme for major acute schemes, the PFI model continues to successfully deliver a number of small- and medium-sized mental health and community schemes. Over 70 such schemes worth approximately £350 million have now reached financial close or are further advanced.
>
> (UK Department of Health Annual Report)

The principal strategy document for resourcing in the NHS in the foreseeable future is the Wanless Report.[77] This report, commissioned by the Treasury rather than the Department of Health, attempts to predict the resource implications of the NHS for the next 20 years:

> Over the next 20 years, the UK will need to devote a substantially larger share of its national income to healthcare, if the vision of the health service in this Report is to be achieved under any of the scenarios. The projections indicate that:
>
> • the growth in spending should be highest in the early years, in order to allow the service to 'catch up', increase activity and deliver higher

quality. As these costs are common across scenarios, early growth is similar in all three scenarios;

- this early growth is at the upper end of what could be sensibly spent, given other resource and capacity constraints, especially the workforce;
- in the later years, the workforce implications of increased activity present a significant challenge and demonstrate the need for skill mix changes and other means of improving productivity; and
- growth in spending in the later years tails off as the service 'keeps up'. But the rate of growth varies between the scenarios and health expenditure accounts for substantially different shares of national income across the scenarios by 2022–23.

The projections for social care show that population changes and the ageing of the population are a much greater cost pressure for social care than for healthcare. The projections do not incorporate the cost of improved quality, and so will underestimate the additional resources required for social care.

The report develops three scenarios in order to model expenditure:

- *solid progress* – people become more engaged in relation to their health: life expectancy rises considerably, health status improves and people have confidence in the primary care system and use it more appropriately. The health service is responsive with high rates of technology uptake and a more efficient use of resources.
- *slow uptake* – there is no change in the level of public engagement: life expectancy rises by the lowest amount in all three scenarios and the health status of the population is constant or deteriorates. The health service is relatively unresponsive with low rates of technology uptake and low productivity.
- *fully engaged* – levels of public engagement in relation to their health are high: life expectancy increases go beyond current forecasts, health status improves dramatically and people are confident in the health system and demand high-quality care. The health service is responsive with high rates of technology uptake, particularly in relation to disease prevention. Use of resources is more efficient.

This report highlights that NHS expenditure will have to increase dramatically (*see* Table 9.2).

**Table 9.2**  Wanless predictions for UK expenditure, 2002–2022[77]

|  | 2002–03 | 2007–08 | 2012–13 | 2017–18 | 2022–23 |
|---|---|---|---|---|---|
| | *Total health spending (% of money GDP)* | | | | |
| Solid progress | 7.7 | 9.4 | 10.5 | 10.9 | 11.1 |
| Slow uptake | 7.7 | 9.5 | 11.0 | 11.9 | 12.5 |
| Fully engaged | 7.7 | 9.4 | 10.3 | 10.6 | 10.6 |

In terms of the implications for the healthcare system, the report indicates that demand will rise dramatically. Only by significant efficiency gains can the UK NHS meet this demand whilst keeping costs within reason. This is reflected in the report's conclusions:[77]

- The Review recommends that the NHS workforce planning bodies should examine the implications of this Review's findings for their projections over the next 20 years.
- It is recommended that future reviews of this type should fully integrate modelling and analysis of health and social care.
- The Review recommends that the National Institute for Clinical Excellence (NICE), in conjunction with similar bodies in the Devolved Administrations, also has a major role to play in examining older technologies and practices which may no longer be appropriate or cost-effective (6.11).
- It will also be important to ensure that recommendations from NICE – particularly its clinical guidelines – are properly integrated with the development of NSFs.
- The Review welcomes the proposed extension of the NSFs to other areas of the NHS.
- It recommends that NSFs should in future include estimates of the resources – in terms of the staff, equipment and other technologies and subsequent cash needs – necessary for their delivery (6.14).
- The Review's projections incorporate a doubling of spending on ICT to fund ambitious targets of the kind set out in the *NHS Information Strategy*. To avoid duplication of effort and resources and to ensure that the benefits of ICT integration across health and social services are achieved, the Review recommends that stringent standards should be set from the centre to ensure that systems across the UK are fully compatible with each other.
- To ensure that resources intended for ICT spending are not diverted to other uses and are used productively, the Review recommends that budgets should be ring-fenced and achievements audited (6.21).
- The Review believes that the scope for greater future cooperation between the NHS and the private sector in the delivery of services should be explored, building on the concordat set out in *The NHS Plan*.
- The Review recommends that there should be a mechanism in place to ensure regular and rigorous independent audit of all healthcare spending and arrangements to ensure it is given maximum publicity (6.37).
- The Review recommends that the Government should examine the merits of employing financial incentives such as those used in Sweden to help reduce the problems of bed blocking.
- The Review believes that the present structure of exemptions for prescription charges is not logical, nor rooted in the principles of the NHS. If related issues are being considered in future, it is recommended that the opportunity should be taken to think through the rationale for the exemption policy (6.75).

- The Review believes that there is an argument for extending out-of-pocket payments for non-clinical services and recommends that they should be kept under review.
- The Review recommends that a more effective partnership between health professionals and the public should be facilitated.
- The Review recommends that the Boards of Strategic Health Authorities (StHAs) should include local patient and business representatives.
- The Review recommends that, as part of improved public engagement, the Department of Health (with StHA involvement) and the Devolved Administrations consider how a greater public appreciation of the cost of common treatments and appointments could best be achieved.
- The Review believes that, as an early step down this road towards better engagement of patients in thinking about the health service, there may be an argument for charging for missed appointments.

The UK NHS has already started to implement these recommendations through, for example, *21st Century IT Support for the NHS*.[78] It remains to be seen if these measures can deliver their objectives, and in turn if these objectives will be perceived as delivering the NHS that patients want.

In the United Kingdom, a larger proportion of healthcare spending is financed by the public sector (84%) than in Canada or Australia (70%). Like the public healthcare insurance scheme of Australia, the NHS is financed mainly through central government general taxation together with an element of national insurance contributions made by employers and employees. User charges account for less than 3% of total NHS financing.

The various waves of reform that swept across the healthcare system in the UK in the course of the 1990s have not significantly altered the ratio between public and private spending as they have concentrated on introducing reforms within the publicly funded system.

Because NHS spending dominates overall expenditures on healthcare in the UK, and because public spending is subject to tight cash limits, the level of spending on healthcare is the subject of intense political debate. One advantage that is often cited for the kind of centralised system that exists in the UK is that it permits a greater degree of overall cost control. This is illustrated by the fact that spending on healthcare in the UK remains low.

Canadian critics encountered by the author argued that although the private sector is a small part of the overall provision, it has a disproportionate effect on the system as a whole. They argue that access to healthcare for those who can afford to pay allows the NHS to get away with access times for the rest of the population that are unacceptable and would 'bring down Governments in Canada'.

# How finance has driven policy in Canada
## Finance and the Canada Health Act

Of the two systems that are characterised as 'public', the UK includes drug costs in its public funding system, Canada generally does not. Over the decade, increasing drug costs in all systems have led to a shift in Canadian expenditure into the private sector. Also, shorter stays in hospital where drug costs in Canada are deemed to be 'medically necessary' have increased the shift in expenditure in to the private sector.

Cam Donaldson, in his evidence to the Canadian Romanow Commission on Health, expresses the differences between the UK and Canada thus:[66]

> Differences also arise with respect to the extent of the two-tier system in different countries. In the UK, everyone is locked into paying for the system. In Canada we pay through our taxes. However, unlike Canada, the UK has no restrictions on private purchase of publicly insured services. That is always portrayed as a great thing about the Canadian system, but one of the paradoxes is that in the UK only 10 per cent to 15 per cent of expenditures come from the private purse: in Canada that figure is 25 per cent. Therefore, what you have here is a different form of the two-tier system. It just covers a different set of services.

In the Canadian context, there remain inconsistencies arising from the definition of 'medically necessary' services:

- Drugs in hospital are publicly funded; once a patient leaves hospital they are not.
- Dentistry services are not considered medically necessary.
- Provinces adopt widely different positions on home- and long-term care (but then so do England and Scotland in the UK!).

This leads to those who argue for an expansion of Medicare to include essential drug costs outside of hospitals:[79]

> ... those countries whose systems most closely approach the principle of single-payer public funding ... also are those that devote the lowest share of GDP to healthcare costs. While Canada strictly respects the single-payer principle with respect to the services covered under the Canada Health Act, the fact that the range of benefits that are covered is relatively narrow means that, in reality, we have a mixed system with a relatively high degree of reliance on private funding. Thus if cost containment is a main objective, there would seem to be a prima-facie case for extending public sector coverage to encompass a broader range of benefits, for example by introducing a system of publicly funded Pharmacare, as suggested by the National Forum on Health.
> (Professor Ake Blomqvist, in evidence to the Romanow Commission)

In 1997, the National Forum on Health report made the following recommendations with regard to reform of drug provision in Canada:[59]

> (a) That pharmaceutical payment policy in Canada be guided by the goals of:
>     – equity of access;
>     – improved prescribing appropriateness; and
>     – cost-containment;

and that to these ends the Canadian Federal–Provincial health insurance system move toward integration of prescription drugs as a fully funded component of publicly funded healthcare.

(b) That the reform process begins with the implementation of comprehensive, population-based drug information systems. These must be publicly run databases, capturing all prescription information regardless of payer, such as now exists in Saskatchewan and British Columbia. They can serve to link physicians, pharmacists, patients and provincial payers, and can then support improved clinical decision making; utilization review; patient information and innovations in reimbursement policies such as extensions of bulk purchasing, the British Columbia reference-based pricing system or developments in 'pharmaceutical benefits management systems' in the United States.

(c) That the Federal Government should undertake to support and assist provincial efforts to manage drug utilization and costs, and avoid initiating any policies that might create impediments to such efforts, while at the same time employing similar management approaches in areas where it has direct responsibility for drug reimbursement, e.g. for Status Indians, Veterans etc.

(d) That as provinces develop experiments with integrated primary healthcare funding envelopes allocated to community-based agencies, budgets for physicians' remuneration be expanded to cover charges for publicly funded prescription drugs (both ingredients and dispensing fees).

(e) That current prohibitions against marketing prescription drugs directly to consumers be maintained, and that such marketing continues to be restricted to health professionals, but that in addition schools that educate health professionals follow the lead of McMaster University Medical School in prohibiting drug marketers from having direct access to students, other than through the director of their program.

(f) That during the up-coming mandatory review of Bill C-91 in 1997, the commitments to increased funding for research made by the pharmaceutical industry at the time of its initial passage be converted into specific required contributions to a fund for health research, broadly defined, at full arm's length from the industry, to be administered by the national research granting agencies and allocated through the normal peer-reviewed granting process.

(g) That while domestic measures to manage drug utilization, improve effectiveness and control costs are pursued with vigour wherever possible, efforts should also be made to initiate concerted action at the international level.

(h) That the Federal Government, Provincial Governments, healthcare providers and private payers (employers, unions and the public) should begin discussions immediately to develop a plan to integrate prescription drugs as a component of publicly funded and administered healthcare as fiscal resources and management technology permit.

The opponents of this approach argue that the cost would be prohibitive, and that although the cost of private provision may be higher in the long term, the impact on the public purse would be disastrous. Even the National Forum on Health qualifies its findings with the phrase 'as fiscal resources and management technology permit'.[59]

Some writers have argued for the introduction of user charges in Canada. This would face massive opposition from the defenders of the Canada Health Act on the basis that it undermines the fundamental principle of universal access to free services. Whilst a consumer of the UK NHS may look enviously at the access of Canadians to essential medical services, the idea that services are truly universal and accessible is simply not sustainable. There are major inequities between rural and urban access. The increasing cost of drugs outside of hospital means that in all areas Canadians are being asked to contribute more to their own healthcare costs.

Supporters of charges argue that they discourage frivolous use and provide a means to limit demand which is otherwise unlimited (see, for example, Charles Wright's lecture).[14] Further, they argue that by diverting funds from charges to fund a national Pharmacare programme, you can provide a more rational set of services within the public programme. They argue that this would facilitate public acceptance of such charges.

Evidence from the UK from prescription charging suggests that the cost of administration, including managing exemptions for the elderly, vulnerable and poor, may significantly reduce the income generated, perhaps even to zero. Therefore, the role of charges becomes to limit demand.

Currently, the Canadians encountered by this author would take a lot of convincing that the reduction in unnecessary demand can be achieved without reducing necessary access. Even in the resource-limited UK system, fees for visiting GPs and thereby gaining access to healthcare have been resisted as being bad for patient health. Not so in Australia …

# Doctor remuneration and primary care reform

A key issue in the financing of Canadian healthcare is the fee-for-service remuneration system for doctors. The fee-for-service system operating in Canada has a fundamental impact on clinician behaviour. From the viewpoint of patients, a valued feature of the fee-for-service remuneration scheme is that it places no significant restrictions on their choice of doctors.

Critics of such a system say that it gives doctors incentives to provide many short visits, but no incentives – in fact disincentives – to fix multiple problems in one visit, or to provide education or counselling activities at the same time. Put simply, doctors who choose to have longer visits, and hence treat fewer patients daily, see in effect their remuneration reduced.

In contrast, primary care in the UK, in other countries such as the Netherlands and in many managed-care plans under American Medicare is provided by general practitioners whose income is based on capitation, working in solo or group practices. Capitation funding, as the name suggests, is a per capita method of compensation. The amount of revenue a GP receives is based on the amount of patients they treat, regardless of the number of visits. One advantage of capitation funding is that it encourages doctors to devote more time to their patients. Capitation, however, carries an incentive to under-service because payment is unrelated to the quantity of services provided. Moreover, a system of capitation that requires individuals to enrol with one particular GP or group of healthcare providers reduces a patient's freedom to choose their own healthcare provider.

One of the attractive properties of a capitation system is that it can be modified to incorporate incentives for primary care physicians to make cost-effective decisions with respect to the use of a wide range of healthcare inputs (drugs, specialists, hospital services, diagnostic testing). Since changes to their remuneration basis in 1990, UK general practitioners receive a mixture of remuneration, including capitation, salary and fee-for-service (for selected items). It has been suggested that this combination of types of payment ensures an effective provision and utilisation of health services.

Finance, however, is not the only factor influencing physician behaviour. The concept of caring for a specific population in the UK is deeply ingrained, although this has been undermined by recent changes in out-of hours care.

However, Canadian researchers have identified that fee-for-service is a major impediment to primary care reform in Canada. According to Cam Donaldson:[66]

> The big difference here compared to many other countries is the remuneration of physicians. To me, this is a great barrier to reforming the system. I personally think that maintaining a fee-for-service form of remuneration is inconsistent with moving to a purchaser–provider model. I do not think that a purchaser–provider model will work with a fee-for-service form of remuneration.

The author observed the development of primary care reform in Ontario with interest and met some of the early adopters of the methods described in the previous chapter. Doctors and their professional associations saw capitation as simply another service in the fee-for-service mechanism. The Provincial Government saw it as a cost-containment mechanism.

The inevitable conclusion from the evaluation report cited in the last chapter is that the reason why the doctors involved were happy was because capitation fees were set high enough to increase their remuneration. The evidence for this politically incorrect conclusion is that the only group of doctors unhappy were those on enhanced fee-for-service, whose income fell.

The implication of this conclusion is that whilst the pilot may be described as a success, it does not provide a basis for rolling out primary care reform to the rest of the province as it would simply be prohibitively expensive in its current form.

# The Federal/Provincial split

Nowhere is the influence of finance more clearly seen in the Canadian system than in the Federal/Provincial split. It has been argued that the role of the Federal Government in financial support of healthcare delivered by the provinces is a constitutional one:[80]

> The spending power in our Constitution is assumed to lie with the Federal Government – to make payments to individuals, to institutions

> or to Provincial Governments, and to make payments even in areas of
> policy that it does not have the constitutional authority to legislate on
> or regulate.... This authority is not written formally into the Constitu-
> tion but has been inferred constitutionally from a number of other
> jurisdictions. This power was core to the development of the welfare
> state in this country and core to the development of health policy.
>
> Under its spending power, the Federal Government can spend money
> that it has raised through taxation or otherwise and set conditions on the
> disposition of funds. The Committee was told that the Federal spending
> power is the basis for transferring funds to the provinces to be used for
> healthcare, and for administering and enforcing the Canada Health Act.
> As we will see below, the Federal Government's role in financially sup-
> porting provincial healthcare delivery is important and has a long history.
>
> (Professor Keith Banting, in evidence to the Romanow Commission)

The Act, which established the original cost-sharing arrangements where there
was a 50–50 split, has been criticised from both ends. From the federal perspective,
it has been argued that it is unpredictable and extremely cumbersome to
administer; whilst from the provinces' perspective it can be perceived to be
inflexible, stifling of innovation and an intrusion into an area of provincial
jurisdiction.

In 1977–78, the 50–50 Federal Provincial cost-sharing arrangements were
replaced by the Established Programs Financing (EPF), a block funding transfer
mechanism that combined federal transfers for hospital services and medical care
with transfers for post-secondary education. The same year, the Federal Government also implemented the Extended Health Care Services Program (EHCSP) to
provide financial assistance to provinces for ambulatory care, nursing home inter-
mediate care, adult residential care and home care. Transfers under the EHCSP
were tied to the EPF block fund. There would no longer be an exact fit between
expenditures and transfers – that is, the Federal Government would make a general transfer that would not be based on what the provinces were spending but
would grow over time with the rate of growth in the economy. The amount transferred would be unrelated to how much the province had actually spent.

This system allowed the Federal Government to control in a very blunt way
their overall healthcare costs. Thus in the early 1990s when Canada went into
recession and healthcare costs peaked at 10% of GDP, contributions to provinces
were reduced further and tensions brought to a head.

In the Budget Speech of February 1995, the Federal Government announced
a new block funding mechanism called the Canada Health and Social Transfer
(CHST) that would cover transfers for healthcare, post-secondary education and
social assistance. The CHST legislation was implemented for the 1996–97 fiscal
year with the coming into force of Bill C-76. Since then, the Federal–Provincial
Fiscal Arrangements Act, which now governs the CHST, has been modified on
five different occasions by the following pieces of legislation: Bill C-31 (1996), Bill
C-28 (1998), Bill C-71 (1999), Bill C-32 (2000) and Bill C-45 (2000). Box 9.1 provides
the details of the various legislative steps for the CHST.[81,82]

The CHST reforms represented a cut in the Federal contribution, but were
balanced by a formula that allowed those contributions to grow in more
prosperous times.

**Box 9.1** A brief history of the CHST[81,82]

**1995**
Budget announced that, starting in 1996–97, EPF replaced by CHST block fund. Meanwhile, for 1995–96, EPF growth set at GDP growth minus 3%.

- CAP frozen at 1994–95 levels for all provinces.
- CHST entitlements set at $26.9 billion for 1996–97 and $25.1 billion for 1997–98.
- CHST entitlements for 1996–97 to be allocated among provinces in the same proportion as combined EPF and CAP entitlements for 1995–96.
- CHST cash transfer to be obtained residually by subtracting the value of the tax transfer from the total CHST entitlement.

**1996**
Budget announced a five-year CHST funding arrangement covering the years 1998–99 to 2002–03.

For 1996–97 and 1997–98, CHST entitlements maintained at $26.9 and $25.1 billion respectively. Then, for 1998–99 and 1999–2000, CHST entitlements fixed at $25.1 billion. For each subsequent fiscal year, through 2002–03, total CHST entitlements set to increase according to an escalator equal to the average GDP growth for the three preceding years, less a predetermined co-efficient (2% in 2000–01, 1.5% in 2001–02 and 1% in 2002–03).

- Guaranteed cash floor of at least $11 billion per year.
- A new allocation formula introduced to reflect differences in provincial population growth and to narrow existing funding disparities, moving halfway to equal per capita entitlements by 2002–03.

**1998**
Legislation passed putting in place a $12.5 billion cash floor under the CHST for the years from 1997–98 to 2002–03 As a result, total CHST entitlements varied directly with the value of tax points, and CHST cash transfer no longer determined residually.

**1999**
Budget announced increased CHST funding of $11.5 billion over five years, and this amount was earmarked specifically for healthcare.

- $8 billion provided through increases to the CHST and $3.5 billion provided through a CHST supplement to give provinces and territories the flexibility to draw down funds over three years as they see fit. One-time cash supplement to be allocated to the provinces on an equal per capita basis.
- The cash floor provision was abolished as the amended legislation provided a level of cash transfer over and above the $12.5 billion limit. Similarly, the escalator used to calculate growth in total CHST entitlements was eliminated since the total entitlement was no more fixed in legislation but varied directly with the cash transfer.

- Changes to the provincial allocation formula accelerated the move to equal per capita CHST by 2001–02.
- CHST legislation extended programme to 2003–04.

**2000**
Budget announced a $2.5 billion increase for the CHST to help provinces and territories fund both post-secondary education and healthcare. These funds were paid into a CHST Supplement Fund and allocated on an equal per capita basis. Provinces can draw down their respective share at any time over the course of four years (2000–01 to 2003–04).

**2001**
The CHST legislation was extended by one year to 2005–06 and the total CHST entitlement was increased by $21.1 billion over a five-year period. The enriched cash transfer is to cover all three fields supported by the CHST, including early child development, and be allocated to the provinces on an equal per capita basis.

Under the new rules, the provincial distribution focuses less on the initial provincial share (based on the former EPF and CAP) and more on the province's demographic weight. As a result, the CHST transfer is moving gradually towards an identical per capita distribution among the provinces. In fact, by 2001–02 all provinces should have received an equal CHST per capita entitlement.

Equal per capita entitlements are to be achieved on a cash and tax basis, not cash alone. The Federal cash contribution, per capita, will still vary from province to province. All equalisation-receiving provinces obtain, as in the past, a per capita CHST cash contribution that is higher than the all-province average. This is due to the fact that they need more Federal cash, per capita, to bring their entitlements to the national average. By contrast, richer provinces will receive more of their Federal support from taxation and less from cash transfers.

Consequently, if the CHST cash component were to be allocated on an equal per capita basis, the total per capita entitlements would be higher for provinces with higher income than for those with lower income because tax points have a higher value in higher income provinces. In the Federal Government's opinion, equal per capita entitlements ensure that all provinces receive equitable Federal support regardless of differences in Provincial Governments' revenues and economic growth rates.

From a patient perspective, the split allows the provinces and the Federal Government to blame each other when resources are deemed to be inadequate. To an outsider, the system seems almost uniquely Canadian. Driven by a strong desire for equity and high quality, the system seems overly complex and bureaucratic to the point where it is puzzling that it works at all. It seems designed to offend and inconvenience all parties equally.

However, in terms of delivering a generally high-quality service to patients at a cost which is by no means prohibitive in comparison to all other systems except possibly the UK, it appears to work rather well. Even in the UK, and even projecting massive improvements in efficiency and management, the Wanless report suggests that the UK will be required to spend more than Canada currently does within ten years.

# How finance has driven policy in Australia

Australia has a national system for the delivery of healthcare which generally covers all permanent residents of Australia. The system is financed largely by general taxes, a proportion of which is raised by an income-related Medicare levy. The proportion of costs met from public funds remains at a level similar to Canada.

There are five major kinds of Commonwealth health funding mechanisms:

- grants to State and Territory Governments under the 1998–2003 Australian Healthcare Agreements to assist with the cost of providing public hospital services
- medical benefits, providing patients with rebates on fees paid to privately practising doctors and optometrists
- pharmaceutical benefits, via the Pharmaceutical Benefits Scheme, providing patients with access to a broad range of subsidised medicines
- Health Programme Grants to government and non-government service providers for a range of health services (for example, radiation oncology [capital component], pathology and primary medical services). Health Programme Grants are used to achieve health policy objectives such as improving access for specific population groups, influencing the growth and distribution of selected and potentially high-cost services, or providing an alternative to fee-for-service arrangements, such as Medicare and the Pharmaceutical Benefits Scheme
- the 30% private health insurance rebate.

In addition to the specific funding mechanisms mentioned above, health services receive part of the general purpose grants provided by the Commonwealth to State and Territory Governments.

When Medicare began in 1984, the levy was introduced as a supplement to other taxation revenue to enable the Government to meet the additional costs of the universal national healthcare system, which were greater than the costs of the more restricted systems that preceded it.

The Medicare levy, which was increased from 1% to 1.25% of taxable income on 1 December 1986, increased to 1.4% on 1 July 1993 and to 1.5% on 1 July 1995.

For 2000–01, the general Medicare levy rate was 1.5% of taxable income. No levy was payable by individuals with income less than $13 807 per year or by families with income less than $23 299, with a further $2140 per year allowed for each child. Single people with incomes above $50 000 and families with incomes above $100 000, with a further $1500 after the first child, who were not covered by private health insurance paid a levy of 2.5% of taxable income, which includes a 1% Medicare levy surcharge.

In a Government decision of 24 May 2000, high-income earners ($50 000 single, $100 000 families) who purchased a high front end deductible (FED) health insurance product were not exempt from the Medicare levy surcharge from 1 July 2000. A high FED costs over $500 for single participants and over $1000 for families.

In 1999–2000, revenue raised from the Medicare levy was approximately 17.5% of total Commonwealth health expenditure and 8.3% of total national health expenditure. The Australian Taxation Office estimated revenue from the Medicare levy to be $4.4 billion in 1999–2000.

Total Commonwealth funding under the 1998–2003 Australian Healthcare Agreements is currently estimated as $31.6 billion over the five years. This is a real increase of around 28% over the life of the Agreements.

In 2000–01, total Commonwealth funding under the Australian Healthcare Agreements was around $6.3 billion. Of this amount:

- $6217m was paid to the States and Territories as healthcare grants, including $134m for quality improvement and enhancement practices in our hospitals, $54m for the implementation of the Second National Mental Health Plan and $30m for the implementation of the National Palliative Care Strategy
- $70m was paid to New South Wales, Victoria, Queensland and Tasmania from the National Health Development Fund
- the remainder was allocated to national initiatives in the areas of mental health, palliative care and case-mix.

For 1999–2000, the preliminary estimate of total expenditure on health services (including both public and private sectors) was $53.7 billion, compared with expenditure of $51.0 billion in the previous year.

This represented an average rate of health services expenditure in 1999–2000 of $2817 per person. In 1999–2000, governments provided more than two-thirds (71%) of the funding for health expenditure, while the remaining 29% was provided by the private sector. Health expenditure in volume terms grew at an average annual rate of 4.0% between 1989–90 and 1999–2000. In 1999–2000, health services expenditure as a proportion of GDP was 8.5%. The ratio was 8.6% in 1998–99, up from 8.4% in 1996–97 and 1997–98.

The evidence has to be that whilst finance appears to have been a factor in driving policy in Australia, the decisions taken have not had the desired effect. The Government has sought to increase private healthcare as a means of controlling cost in the public sector.

Figure 9.3 shows that whilst total expenditure peaked in 1998, reductions since have been in the private sector and the public expenditure has continued to grow.

## Discussion

Finance is clearly a major driver in health policy. However, there are a number of paradoxes and misunderstandings that characterise the relationship, which means that the basic premise that a modern healthcare system cannot be funded from the public purse is too simple a view to be applied uncritically:

- The healthcare reforms of the 1990s were introduced as a response to apparently accelerating healthcare costs attributed to an ageing population and increasingly

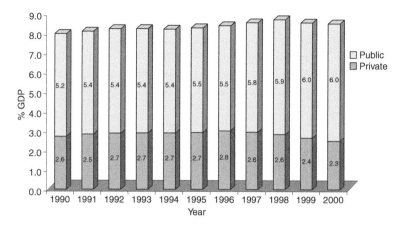

**Figure 9.3**   % GDP spent on healthcare in Australia 1990–2000, split by public/private contribution.

high technology treatments. In reality, it was nations' ability to pay that was the problem. This was caused by a global recession.

• There is much evidence that private provision costs more than public provision. This has been argued in both the Canadian and Australian contexts which represent opposing poles with regard to the provision of private services.

• One of the costs that is accelerating most quickly is drug costs. However, the increased use of modern drugs produces significant savings by removing patients from hospital care much more quickly or in some cases preventing the need for hospital admission completely. No system had the means to show how the increasing costs on the one hand were offset by preventative costs.

• If drug costs are the major concern in increasing costs and public provision is demonstrably the cheaper option, it makes no sense for Canadians to exclude drugs from their public system.

• The commitment to private healthcare in Australia has had only one demonstrable effect: to increase the proportional and absolute contribution from public funds.

Overall, policy appears to be driven more by politicians' beliefs about what will save money rather than evidence. We shall return to this theme in Chapter 11.

# CHAPTER 10

# Driver 2: scandals

## Introduction

In the UK and to a lesser extent in Canada and Australia, healthcare policy has been driven by a need to respond to a series of scandals which have become public in recent years, although they relate to events from an earlier period.

## Scandals in the UK

There has been a significant number of adverse incidents in the UK NHS in recent years. We shall consider the three most significant incidents:

- Bristol paediatric cardiology
- Alder Hey organ retention
- Dr Harold Shipman.

The events in Bristol, which date back to the 1980s, were concerned with the deaths of children undergoing cardiac surgery.[83] Between 1988 and 1995 Mr Janardan Dhasmana, a heart surgeon at the Bristol Royal Infirmary (BRI), one of nine centres in the UK specialising in children's heart surgery, carried out 38 arterial switch operations – and 20 of the young patients died. Between 1990 and 1994, heart surgeon Mr James Wisheart performed 15 atrio-ventricular septal defect (ASVD) operations. A total of nine of the young patients died.

In 1991, Dr John Roylance was appointed Chief Executive of the United Bristol Healthcare NHS Trust, and in the following year Mr Wisheart was appointed Medical Director of the hospital. In 1995, Mr Wisheart stopped operating on children and concentrated on adult heart surgery. In the same year, Dr Roylance retired.

In 1988, Dr Stephen Bolsin, a consultant anaesthetist, joined the BRI. He noticed that children's heart operations lasted up to three times as long as in other hospitals and that youngsters were dying from relatively routine operations.

In 1990 Dr Bolsin had written to the then head of the district health authority, later to be BRI Chief Executive, to raise his concerns about what seemed to be a higher than average death rate for newly born babies undergoing cardiac surgery. His allegations against the head of his cardiac unit, James Wisheart, were dismissed and Dr Bolsin claims the surgeon then threatened to ruin his career prospects should he continue to pursue the matter. He was left with little choice but to carry out his own audit of results. Fortunately, he was in charge of audit for the Royal College of Anaesthetists.

Bolsin soon confirmed that, for one particular hole-in-the-heart procedure, nine out of 12 of Mr Wisheart's patients had died – a figure far higher than the national average. He was also very concerned about the other surgeon, Janardan Dhasmana's record for a complex operation known as 'the switch'. Over the period in question Dhasmana carried out 38 operations with 20 deaths.

The last operation took place in January 1995. The night before, an extraordinary meeting of the cardiac team took place. Every doctor, except Dr Bolsin, agreed the operation should go ahead. But concerns about the whole switch programme had spread outside the hospital because Dr Bolsin had contacted a key official from the Department of Health.

That evening Dr John Roylance had a phone call at home from the official, who expressed worries about the operation going ahead. The former Chief Executive said that, although he was a doctor, he could not intervene over the clinical judgement of the doctors directly involved. The operation went ahead and the patient died. At this point Dr Bolsin went to the media.

In 1996, parents wrote to the General Medical Council (GMC), the doctors' regulatory body, asking for an investigation into the professional conduct of Mr Wisheart, Dr Roylance and Mr Dhasmana. Mr Wisheart suspended all his surgery and stepped down as Medical Director, and in the following year he retired. In June 1998 the GMC found Mr Wisheart, Dr Roylance and Mr Dhasmana guilty of serious professional misconduct. Mr Wisheart and Dr Roylance were struck off the Register and Mr Dhasmana was banned from operating on children for three years. Dr Roylance decided to appeal against the GMC ruling.

The GMC issued new guidelines telling doctors how and when they should report a colleague whose performance they thought was putting patient safety at risk.

Following this, the then Health Secretary, Frank Dobson, ordered an inquiry into the heart surgery service at Bristol Royal Infirmary:[84]

> To inquire into the management of the care of children receiving complex cardiac surgical services at the Bristol Royal Infirmary between 1984 and 1995 and relevant related issues; to make findings as to the adequacy of the services provided; to establish what action was taken both within and outside the hospital to deal with concerns raised about the surgery and to identify any failure to take appropriate action promptly; to reach conclusions from these events and to make recommendations which could help to secure high-quality care across the NHS.
>
> (Secretary of State for Health, Frank Dobson,
> June 1998, Speech to Parliament)

Even before the inquiry started, the Department of Health announced a raft of measures to ensure high standards in the NHS, including:

- the use of NICE to set guidelines for best practice
- a Commission for Health Improvement (CHI) to ensure that practitioners met the standards set by NICE
- plans that gave patients a say in doctors' merit awards – payments that could double a consultant's earnings. (This came about after it emerged that Mr Wisheart had received an A merit award worth £50 000 a year)
- the publication of league tables of the death rates at hospitals.

Mr Dhasmana was sacked by BRI, but decided to appeal, backed by a group of former patients and relatives.

A week before the inquiry was due to start preliminary hearings at the end of October, the Senate of Surgery issued proposals to ensure that doctors monitored their own performance and were not allowed to carry out procedures that were beyond their competence. It also proposed 'rapid response teams' of specialists to review surgery at hospitals where death rates were unacceptably high. Under the proposals, consultants would have to undergo regular appraisals to establish that they were still fit to practise. In February 1999, doctors at the GMC voted that they should be demoted or even struck off if they do not pass regular tests on their skills.

Dr John Roylance appealed to the Privy Council to have the GMC's decision to strike him off the Medical Register overturned.

Meanwhile, parents' groups were angered as it emerged that the hospital had retained the organs of some dead babies. The hospital said it was standard practice to remove organs for post-mortems and consent was not a legal requirement. However, the Secretary of State said this was disturbing and the inquiry needed to look into the issue.

On the eve of full hearings at the public inquiry, Mr Dhasmana, who lost the appeal against his sacking, said he planned to take his former employers before an industrial tribunal.

The public inquiry started in Bristol in May 1999 and reported in July 2001. The 198 recommendations[83] covered the following areas:

- respect and honesty
- a health service which is well led
- competent healthcare professionals
- the safety of care
- care of an appropriate standard
- public involvement through empowerment
- the care of children.

Some of the key recommendations were:

1 In a patient-centred healthcare service patients must be involved, wherever possible, in decisions about their treatment and care.

12 Patients must be given such information as enables them to participate in their care.

24 The process of informing the patient and obtaining consent to a course of treatment should be regarded as a process and not a one-off event consisting of obtaining a patient's signature on a form.

34 When things go wrong, patients are entitled to receive an acknowledgement, an explanation and an apology.

41 The various bodies whose purpose it is to assure the quality of care in the NHS (for example, CHI and NICE) and the competence of healthcare professionals (for example, the GMC and the Nursing and Midwifery Council) must themselves be independent of, and at arm's length from, the Department of Health.

69 Regulation of healthcare professionals is not just about disciplinary matters. It should be understood as encapsulating all of the systems

which combine to assure the competence of healthcare professionals: education, registration, training, continuous professional development and revalidation as well as disciplinary matters.

88 Periodic revalidation, whereby healthcare professionals demonstrate that they remain fit to practise in their chosen profession, should be compulsory for all healthcare professionals. The requirement to participate in periodic revalidation should be included in the contract of employment.

132 One body should be responsible for validating and revalidating NHS trusts and primary care trusts. This body should be CHI, suitably structured so as to give it the necessary independence and authority. Other bodies (for example the NHS Litigation Authority) which are currently concerned with setting and requiring compliance with those generic standards which should fall within the authority of CHI, should carry out their role in this respect under the authority of, and answerable to, CHI.

191 Healthcare professionals should be honest and truthful with parents in discussing their child's condition, possible treatment and the possible outcome.

The major impact of Bristol is that it undermined the perceived infallibility of doctors and hospital consultants in particular. This was summed up in a *BMJ* editorial:[85]

> The Bristol case, in which judgment was passed last week, will probably prove much more important to the future of healthcare in Britain than the reforms suggested in the White Papers. Reorganisations of the NHS come round with monotonous regularity, but changes on the wards and in surgeries are slow and often unrelated to the passing political rhetoric. In contrast, the Bristol case is a once-in-a-lifetime drama that has held the attention of doctors and patients in a way that a White Paper can never hope to match. The case has thrown up a long list of important issues (see box) that British medicine will take years to address. At the heart of the tragedy, which has been Shakespearean in its scale and structure, is, as the GMC said, 'the trust that patients place in their doctors'. That trust will never be the same again, but that will be a good thing if we move to an active rather than a passive trust, where doctors share uncertainty.
>
> (Richard Smith)

In the Bristol inquiry, one of the major issues for parents was the retention of organs for post-mortem. One parent quoted in the final report stated that:[83]

> We would have liked it if even perhaps a year or so, but certainly a few months before, there had been what I describe as just a routine appointment with a liaison counsellor and that particular person, as a matter of routine, if they had just said to us, 'It is my job, my job description to go through this with you, Mr.... It is not because of Bethan's particular case, I have to do this with every patient.' If they had that expectation to deliver certain information such as what bereavement facilities were

available in the unfortunate event of death, what was entailed with post-mortem, what that exactly was, so that we were clear....

The way that we would have liked it in our circumstances is if it had been conveyed before death, and I say 'before death' because if it had been done in a routine manner; what was the procedure for complaints, what the line of communication was, to whom we should go, what the facilities were as regards bereavement, what post-mortem meant, but also, especially about the retention of organs. I think we would have perceived it better if it had been a few months or even a year or so before the operation; not just before the operation, but a few months before.

This matter came to a head when it emerged that many children's organs had been retained at the Alder Hey Children's Hospital in Liverpool. The scandal at Alder Hey emerged almost accidentally when heart specialist, Professor Robert Anderson, revealed at the Bristol inquiry that a store of children's hearts was kept at Alder Hey.

It became apparent that organ harvesting at Alder Hey had been such an established practice that, even parents whose children had died decades ago, found that organs had been removed before the bodies were released to the families. It was shown that, even when the hospital told parents that organs were missing from the bodies of their dead children, some parents were still not given the whole truth. In some cases, parents had organs returned to them for burial only to require another funeral just months later when another organ or piece of tissue was returned. In total 2080 children's hearts and the organs of more than 800 children were kept at Alder Hey, along with 400 fetuses collected from hospitals across the region.

Professor Dick van Velzen, the pathologist at the centre of the Alder Hey scandal, admitted using some organs for research purposes without the permission of the coroner or the consent of parents. He blamed the hospital for the practice of organ stripping, claiming that he removed and stored the organs of 845 children because he did not have the resources from the hospital to carry out detailed post-mortems and that he had always hoped to complete them one day.

Just a month after the revelation of the organ retention in October 1999, the then Health Secretary, Frank Dobson, ordered an investigation into the retention of body parts for medical research. Mr Dobson said the Department of Health would be working closely with the Royal College of Pathologists to produce new guidelines clarifying what relatives have agreed to when they give permission for a post-mortem.

The new guidelines came out in March 2000 and called for full consent from relatives before a post-mortem examination is carried out, and before organs and tissues are retained, either to determine the cause of death or for medical research.

The British Medical Association (BMA) issued its own guidance in October 2000, telling doctors to be more aware of relatives' feelings when asking to keep body tissues.

In December 1999, the Government announced that it would be holding a public inquiry following the revelations that other hospitals around Britain had also been retaining organs. The hospital [Alder Hey] also launched its own internal investigation and the case was reported to the GMC.

In January 2001, Professor Liam Donaldson, the Chief Medical Officer, told distressed parents that he would be backing a change in the law to ensure that hospitals could never again retain organs without permission.

The Human Tissue Act (1961) makes it clear that doctors cannot make a decision themselves on whether to keep organs unless the patient is a child who has died after a pregnancy lasting less than 24 weeks. Otherwise they must make reasonable enquiries of parents and relatives.

Coroners in England, Wales and Northern Ireland have the power to authorise a special post-mortem into a body where there is some doubt as to the cause of death.

The report into Alder Hey made many recommendations, of which the key points were:[86]

- Serious incident procedures should be developed and put in place.
- Clinicians requesting a hospital post-mortem examination after the Coroner has declined to authorise an examination shall make it clear to the next of kin that there is no compulsion remaining for such an examination.
- Clinicians shall explain the contents and implications of a Coroner's post-mortem report to the next of kin as if the examination had been carried out as a hospital post-mortem examination on their own recommendation.
- In the preceding Chapter we concluded that fully informed consent is required and nothing less. Fully informed consent must be freely given without imposition of pressure. It is the application of basic principles of respect for the person, their welfare and wishes.
- Comprehensive information is required to obtain a valid consent. Parents must be informed of the identity of each organ to be retained and the purpose for which it is to be used. Dr Peart, a Consultant Paediatric Cardiologist at Alder Hey, accepts that consent forms must be specific about every organ to be retained. Blanket consent is inadequate for organs but is worthy of further consideration with regard to the retention of small tissue samples for diagnostic purposes, medical education and research.
- Fully informed consent means that a person must have all the information required to form a final decision. It is not enough for clinicians to tell the next of kin that they would like to examine the body after death and this might involve taking some tissue. The next of kin need to understand what is involved in a post-mortem examination, including a description of whole body systems, removal of the brain and the steps necessary to remove various organs, no matter how distasteful the giving of this information might be to the clinician concerned.

The final scandal to emerge around this time was that of Dr Harold Shipman, a GP who was convicted of killing 15 patients and who is believed to have killed approximately 300.

In 1974, Dr Harold Shipman became an assistant general practitioner and then a general practitioner principal at Todmorden Group Practice in the Abraham Ormerod Medical Centre in Todmorden, on the Lancashire–West Yorkshire border.

A year later it was discovered that large quantities of controlled drugs were being prescribed by Dr Shipman. He underwent treatment at The Retreat, a psychiatric centre in York, from early October to late December.

During 1976, Dr Shipman was convicted at Halifax Magistrates Court of dishonestly obtaining drugs, forgery of NHS prescriptions and unlawful possession of pethidine. He was fined on each charge and ordered to pay compensation to the Family Practitioner Committee. During this year Dr Shipman worked as a clinical medical officer in south west Durham.

In 1977, Dr Shipman joined Donneybrook House Group Practice in Hyde, Cheshire as a general practitioner, and in 1992 he moved to The Surgery, 21 Market Street, Hyde and set up as a single-handed GP.

In March 1998, a local GP reported concerns to the Coroner about the excess number of deaths among Shipman's patients. Following further investigations, in September Shipman was arrested by the Greater Manchester police.

On 31 January 2000, the jury at Preston Crown Court returned guilty verdicts against Shipman on 15 counts of murder and one of forgery of a will.

On 1 February 2000, the Secretary of State for Health announced an inquiry into the case under Section 2 of the National Health Service Act 1977. In March, the terms of reference were published for the independent inquiry under the chairmanship of Lord Laming of Tewin. The inquiry was to sit in private but its report would be made public.

A group of relatives and friends of known or suspected victims of Shipman, plus several media groups, applied to the High Court for judicial review of the Secretary of State's decision. In July, those applications succeeded and the Laming Inquiry was disbanded. In September, the Secretary of State for Health announced that a public inquiry would be held under the Tribunals of Inquiry (Evidence) Act 1921, and in December, Dame Janet Smith DBE, a High Court judge, was invited to become chairman of the inquiry.

This inquiry gave its interim report in 2001:[87]

> I have found that Shipman committed serious criminal offences throughout his professional career. From 1974, he regularly obtained controlled drugs by illicit means. In August 1974, he unlawfully administered an opiate, probably pethidine, to Mrs Elaine Oswald, causing her to suffer respiratory arrest and putting her life at risk. He first killed a patient, Mrs Eva Lyons, in March 1975. She was suffering from cancer and was terminally ill. Shipman gave her a lethal overdose and hastened her death. In the 24 years during which Shipman worked as a doctor, I have found that, in addition to the 15 patients of whose murder he was convicted, he killed 200 patients. In a further 45 cases there is real cause to suspect that Shipman might have killed the patient. In 38 cases, I have been unable to reach a conclusion of any kind due to the insufficiency of evidence. These deaths occurred mainly in the early years of Shipman's career, for which there are few written records. I regret that the families of these patients will be left in a state of uncertainty. Shipman's last victim was Mrs Kathleen Grundy, who died on 24th June 1998. In 210 of the cases in which I have written a decision, I have found that the death was certainly or probably natural.
>
> (Dame Janet Smith, Chair, Shipman Inquiry)

The final report with recommendations for the future is as yet unpublished at the time of writing. However, it is clear that the intention is to recommend monitoring systems to protect patients:

> It is deeply disturbing that Shipman's killing of his patients did not arouse suspicion for so many years. The systems which should have safeguarded his patients against his misconduct, or at least detected misconduct when it occurred, failed to operate satisfactorily. The esteem in which Shipman was held ensured that very few relatives felt any real sense of disquiet about the circumstances of the victims' deaths. Those who did harbour private suspicions felt unable to report their concerns. It was not until March 1998 that any fellow professional felt sufficiently con-cerned to make a report to the coroner. Unfortunately, Dr Linda Reynolds' report of 24th March 1998 came to nought. Had it not been for Shipman's grossly incompetent forgery of Mrs Grundy's will, it is by no means clear that his crimes would ever have been detected.

The effect of these scandals has been to move the quality agenda within the NHS strongly towards the systematic view of quality, designed to prevent catastrophic failure rather than to achieve routine improvements in patient care.

Consider the following extract from *The New NHS* White Paper in 1997, regard-ing performance measurement:[15]

> The new framework will demonstrate progress on the overall goals of the NHS, on the key steps the NHS must take to deliver those goals and on the outcomes it is achieving. It will have six dimensions:
>
> **Health improvement**
> To reflect the overall aim of improving the general health of the popu-lation, which is influenced by many factors, reaching well beyond the NHS. For example, changes in rates of premature death, reflecting social and economic factors as well as healthcare.
>
> **Fair access**
> To recognise that the NHS contribution must begin by offering fair access to health services in relation to people's needs, irrespective of geography, class, ethnicity, age or sex. For example, ensuring that black and minority ethnic groups are not disadvantaged in terms of access to services.
>
> **Effective delivery of appropriate healthcare**
> To recognise that fair access must be to care that is effective, appro-priate and timely, and complies with agreed standards. For example, increasing provision of treatments proven to bring benefit such as hip replacements, provision of rehabilitation at the point when it can offer most benefit, sustained delivery of health and social care to those with long-term needs, and reducing inappropriate treatments.
>
> **Efficiency**
> The way in which the NHS uses its resources to achieve value for money. For example, length of hospital stay; day surgery rates; unit costs;

labour productivity; management overheads; capital productivity. The NHS will be able to assess the impact it has made through offering *fair access* to *effective* care, *efficiently* delivered, by two further measures:

### Patient/carer experience

Through measuring the way in which patients and carers view the quality of the treatment and care that they receive, ensuring the NHS is sensitive to individual needs. For example, new national patient survey; new NHS Charter.

### Health outcomes of NHS care

And finally, through assessing the direct contribution of NHS care to improvements in overall health, completing the circle back to the overarching goal of improved health. For example, trends in infectious diseases for which immunisation programmes are available.

Compare that with *The NHS Plan* in 2001:[74]

> **1.21** People will have the reassurance that the NHS is adopting high standards and striving continuously to improve the quality of its care. Every hospital, primary and community care service and nursing home will issue an annual prospectus setting out its standards, performance and the views of its patients. The funding received by local NHS organisations will be based in part on the results of regular patient surveys. **1.22** National standards for treating all the major conditions will have been established. Appropriate drugs and treatments which are shown to be clinically and cost-effective will be in use in every part of the country. Doctors, therapists and nurses will increasingly work to standard protocols. There will be independent inspection of NHS organisations.

The impact of these scandals may be seen in:

* rigid national standards
* external independent inspections.

Whilst the patient is being empowered, the role and independence of the clinicians have been eroded. For the vast majority of competent dedicated staff, these changes may result in more bureaucracy and a reduction in motivation.

   The organisation that is driving quality assurance is the Commission for Health Improvement, established in April 2000. Its purpose is described as follows:[88]

> The Commission for Health Improvement (CHI) was established to improve the quality of patient care in the NHS. It does this by reviewing the care provided by the NHS in England and Wales (Scotland has its own regulatory body, the Clinical Standards Board). CHI aims to address unacceptable variations in NHS patient care by identifying both notable practice and areas where care could be improved. CHI has six operating principles that underpin all of its work:
>
> * The patient's experience is at the heart of CHI's work.

- CHI will be independent, rigorous and fair.
- CHI's approach is developmental and will support the NHS to continuously improve.
- CHI's work will be based on the best available evidence and focus on improvement.
- CHI will be open and accessible.
- CHI will apply the same standards of continuous improvement to itself that it expects of others.

The CHI monitors patient care and seeks to improve quality by carrying out clinical governance reviews. It visits all NHS organisations (including acute trusts, ambulance trusts, general practices, mental health trusts, primary care trusts and their equivalent in Wales) in England and Wales on a continuous programme.

The CHI states that effective clinical governance should guarantee that:

- patient services continue to improve
- staff treat patients courteously and involve them in decisions about their care
- patients have all the information they need about their care
- health professionals are up to date in their practices
- health professionals are supervised
- clinical errors are prevented wherever possible.

It has a number of other roles:

- It monitors and reviews how the NHS meets the recommendations of National Service Frameworks and NICE guidelines. NSFs make recommendations about the quality of service that patients should expect from a specific area of healthcare. The first CHI national study report into cancer care in England and Wales was published in December 2001.[88] The next study, which will look at implementation of the NSF for Coronary Heart Disease, will be published in 2004.
- It investigates serious service failures in the NHS. All requests for investigations either from the Secretary of State for Health, the National Assembly for Wales (NAW) or members of the public will be carefully considered. The CHI does not duplicate work carried out as part of the NHS complaints system. It will only investigate issues if there are lessons to be learned across the NHS.

Finally, CHI is charged with leading, reviewing and assisting NHS healthcare improvement and aims to collect and share notable practice in the NHS.

The goals of the CHI may be divided into patient-centred goals and professional-centred goals. It seeks to review practice through a review process. Since early 2002, the review has been a 17-week process. Every review team includes a NHS doctor, nurse, professional allied to medicine or a pharmacist or therapist, a lay member and a manager.

Reviews into health authorities and the bodies they cover also include a GP in the review team. A CHI review manager leads and manages the team for the duration of the review (*see* Box 10.1).

This methodology is not new. It is similar to that employed by OFSTED in the inspection of schools and the QAA in universities for approximately ten years. The criticism that has been directed against such reviews is that it is hard to

**Box 10.1**   The CHI review process

**Preparation stage: three months prior to visit**
*Requests for information*
The CHI will request various types of data and reports to prepare for its site visit. This information is analysed and assists in identifying specific areas the review team will look at during its visit. It is essential to the success of the review and requires the NHS organisation to do some preparatory work.

NHS organisations collect data and information and send these to the CHI within the three-month period.

To ensure that the process runs as smoothly as possible, the Trust is asked to nominate a member of staff to coordinate the review process on their behalf and act as a focal point. This will be the Trust coordinator.

*Requests for local opinion*
The CHI will actively seek the opinions of patients, staff, relatives of patients and local organisations interested in the NHS organisation being reviewed. This information will help draw together themes of public opinion and will be considered as part of the review.

Early in the review process, the trust coordinator may wish to start collating a list of stakeholder names, addresses and contact numbers and possible non-hospital-based, accessible stakeholder meeting venues.

*Open lines of communication*
The CHI will be as open and accessible as possible to ensure a successful review process. It will meet with the management teams at the organisation being reviewed to explain the review process and answer questions.

**The review proper**
*Week 1*
- Analysis of data and information begins.
- CHI holds first meeting with NHS organisation.
- CHI asks that the following people are invited to the meeting:
  – Chief Executive
  – the Trust's clinical governance lead
  – the nominated Trust coordinator
  – Medical Director
  – Director of Nursing
  – Director(s) responsible for allied health professionals and pharmacists
  – Head of Communications
  – Up to four people from CHI will attend the meeting, including the Review Manager and Communications Officer.

*Week 4*
- Stakeholder events.

*Week six*
- CHI team and reviewers present emerging key themes to the NHS organisation.
- NHS organisation presents its view of its clinical governance capabilities to CHI.

*Week 8*
- CHI review team at NHS organisation for week-long visit.
- The team of CHI reviewers spend about one week visiting the site with some weekend and night observations.
- The team meets with clinicians, managers and other staff to collect information about clinical governance in the organisation. Individuals are not named in the report. The review team will observe patients and staff together, but not in operating theatres or consultation/treatment rooms.
- CHI feeds back its findings to the NHS organisation.
- After the visit, the review team drafts a report of their findings. The report is discussed with the NHS organisation being reviewed which comments on its factual accuracy.

*Week 17*
- The final summary and report is published and is available to the public and on CHI's website. It contains CHI's key findings and identifies best practice as well as areas for improvement.

*Follow-up*
In the final stages of the review process, the NHS organisation will begin to work on its action plan. After the publication of the report, CHI will assist the organisation to set objectives to take forward improvements needed. The local regional office or the National Assembly for Wales takes a vital role in approving the action plan and is responsible for ensuring it is implemented.

capture the reality of the patient experience in a snapshot. Such reviews emphasise processes and documentation.

To look at a CHI review, consider the Northumbria NHS Trust review, chosen as the first after the CHI streamlined its processes in 2002.[88]

The CHI process itself creates an artificial situation. Staff are motivated to show the Trust in the best possible light. This is emphasised by a grade assigned on a scale from I to IV. On the basis of the evidence collected, the CHI's reviewers assess each component of clinical governance using this four-point scale:

I   **Little or no progress** at strategic and planning levels or at operational level.
II  **Worthwhile progress and development** at strategic and planning levels or at operational level, but not at both.
III **Good strategic grasp and substantial implementation** – alignment of activity and development across the strategic and planning levels and operational levels of the Trust.

IV **Excellence** – coordinated activity and development across the organisation and with partner organisations in the local health economy that demonstrably lead to improvement. Clarity about the next stage of clinical governance development.

In essence, this is a process strongly rooted in the systemic view of quality, and has much in common with the 1987 ISO 9000 series of quality management standards. These have been widely criticised for producing systems designed to perform well under a specific review methodology rather than a more general improvement culture. Inevitably, much of the judgement is based upon documentation rather than detailed evaluation of the reality of operation.

Although much is made in the CHI documentation of the patient-centeredness of the process, in reality the major focus here is around the processes that impact upon patient care and the ability of the trust to manage them.

# Scandals in Canada

In a bizarre and tragic coincidence, Canada has experienced its own parallel scandal to the Bristol case in Winnipeg, Manitoba.[89] Twelve infants and children died during or after cardiac surgery between February and December of 1994. During that period, the overall cardiac surgery in-hospital mortality rate was 15%, in contrast to that at the Hospital for Sick Children (Toronto) where the overall rate was 4.5%. The mortality rate in Winnipeg for children under one year of age was 29%, and was described by Drs Williams and Roy in their review report as 'clearly excessive', in contrast to Toronto's rate of 11%.

In 1982, Dr George Collins became the section head of paediatric cardiology in Winnipeg at the Health Sciences Center (HSC). Collins was also given the mandate to develop what came to be known as the Variety Children's Heart Centre (VCHC) and served as the VCHC's first Medical Director.

The VCHC was established and expanded under Dr Collins to a team of four paediatric cardiologists. However, between 1990 and 1993 all four cardiologists left and due to financial restrictions their positions were not refilled.

In April 1993, Collins gave notice of his intention to leave at the end of six months. Whilst he later said that he had always planned to leave Winnipeg for other opportunities after ten years, his letter explaining his resignation also spoke of his frustrations as Medical Director of the VCHC and with the manner in which the hospital and the Government of Manitoba were addressing issues related to paediatric cardiac surgery in the province. In his letter of resignation, Collins questioned the commitment of both the HSC and the Government to provide the programme with sufficient support for it to achieve its objectives.

At about the same time as Collins left Winnipeg, the solo paediatric cardiac surgeon also left. Concerns were then raised that it would be difficult to attract a capable candidate for paediatric cardiac surgery to Winnipeg and it would be even more difficult to retain such a candidate. However, a seemingly well-qualified individual was found. He was a US-trained doctor who had undergone a portion of his training in Canada. His last post was as one of five residents (senior registrars) at one of the world's leading centres for such surgery, Boston Children's Hospital, which is affiliated with Harvard University.

Dr Odim was appointed in November 1993. However, his recruitment and hiring process appears to have been flawed:[89]

> No one spoke with the people who had been most recently involved in Odim's training at Boston. Considering Mayer's very lukewarm assessment of Odim's surgical skills, it is conceivable that Odim might not have been hired had that type of information been in the hands of those making the hiring decisions in Winnipeg in 1994. The failure to watch and observe Odim actually performing surgery, or to speak with anyone who had recently performed surgery with him, provided only an incomplete impression of Odim's surgical abilities and his ability to get along with other personnel in the operating room.

Odim took up his duties on 14 February 1994, and performed his first operation on 28 February. The case proceeded smoothly and team members were encouraged by its success. Over the year, over 70 children underwent paediatric cardiac surgery and many of those cases passed without any significant incident. By March he was performing very complex operations. From then until May that year, it would appear that only one paediatric cardiac surgery patient was referred out of province, in contrast with previous practice. Previously, newly appointed surgeons had taken on complex cases more gradually. At this stage, problems were already emerging:

- lack of an orientation programme for Dr Odim
- lack of attention to team building
- Dr Odim's treatment of nurses and response to advice offered
- Dr Odim's failure to take advantage of opportunities offered
- Dr Odim's expressed concern with the number of anaesthetists or the limitations of the intensive care unit (ICU) wards
- failure by either Dr Odim or the paediatric cardiologist to refer complex cases outside of province, in line with previous practice.

By May, major problems were apparent:[89]

> On Monday, May 16, 1994, the paediatric anaesthesia section met. It was at this meeting that the section voted to take the extraordinary step of withdrawing services to paediatric cardiac surgery. Swartz, McNeill, Wong and Reimer outlined their concerns with the program. They were concerned about morbidity and mortality, the apparent lack of monitoring and the deteriorating relations among team members. According to McNeill, the members of the section who did not give anaesthetics for open cardiac procedures all expressed their support for the four who did.

The result was that the anaesthetists suspended their services with immediate effect until a review could be undertaken. A review committee was created known as the Paediatric Cardiac Review Team, or the Wiseman Committee, and met for the first time on 18 May. In retrospect, however, the committee may have been established too quickly as some important matters were not addressed. Because the committee was created outside existing processes, it lacked a clear structure and rules of procedure. It was not clear what authority the committee had to change existing procedures or seek advice from outside experts.

At that meeting, it was agreed that the anaesthetists would participate in less-complex, low-risk open-heart cases but that they would not participate in cases of higher risk until the review was complete.

The review was completed by September 1994, and the members of the paediatric cardiac surgery team prepared to return to a fully operational programme. Some team members still harboured significant concerns about the programme's ability to provide appropriate care for patients with heart defects of high complexity. As was the case before the original showdown of 16 May, that concern rested almost exclusively with the nurses and the anaesthetists. The head of anaesthesia met with the paediatric cardiac anaesthetists. He wanted reassurances from them that, since the programme would be returning to full service, the paediatric cardiac anaesthetists would be full participants. The nature and tone of the discussion reflected the anaesthetists' lack of support for the decision to return the programme to full activity.

By the end of September, many of the nurses were once more disturbed and distressed by the operation of the programme. The problems that confronted the nurses do not reflect a lack of professional responsibility on their part; rather, they appear to reflect the historically subordinate role that the nursing profession has played in our healthcare system. In this case, none of the persons involved actually went outside the processes available to address the concerns they had.

In December, disquiet was once again reaching the more senior members of the hospital. The neonatal staff were losing confidence in the paediatric cardiac surgery programme. They spoke both of the deaths of patients and the extended stays in ICU of those infants who survived surgery. Others brought up concerns with the length of bypass times and problems with pacemakers. It became apparent that the neonatologists had lost confidence in the programme and were reluctant to refer even emergency cases to it. A decision was made that such cases would, for the immediate future, be referred out of province. Since no elective operations were scheduled for the Christmas period, this meant that the programme was temporarily inactive.

A review was again ordered and after an attempt to hold an internal review failed, two outside experts from Toronto were brought in to carry it out.

On 25 January 1995, the external reviewers met from 0730 hours to 1900 hours with individuals involved in the programme. On the other hand, the nurses were not informed of the appointment of these reviewers and they were not at that time asked to prepare any written submissions. From their itinerary, while it would appear that they met with operating-room nurses, it does not appear that the reviewers spoke with any of the neonatal ICU or paediatric ICU nurses.

The review report listed ten conclusions, including:

- that there was evidence to question Odim's technical competence
- that Odim might have been judged unfairly since he had attempted to adopt the HSC's methods rather than import his own preferences
- that the programme had been poorly supported by the HSC from the outset.

The reviewers specifically stated that their report 'neither exonerates nor condemns the present surgeon'.

On 14 February 1995, the HSC issued a news release that announced a further 'intensive six-month review' and confirmed that:

> This decision was made because patient outcomes have not achieved standards which the hospital hoped for when the program was reintroduced in February 1994.

The news release concluded with the statement that, from that point, patients would be referred out of province. After this no further paediatric cardiac surgery was carried out in Manitoba.

The families of the 12 children who had died in 1994 mostly heard about the shutdown through the media. The news shocked and distressed them. They demanded a public inquiry.

On 5 March 1995, following a meeting with the Minister of Justice and other representatives of the Department of Justice, the Chief Medical Examiner for the Province of Manitoba ordered that an inquest be held into the deaths of the 12 children. He directed that one inquest be convened to investigate all the 1994 deaths. The Minister of Justice declined to appoint a public inquiry, indicating that the matter might be reconsidered once the inquest had reported.

The inquest report concludes:[89]

> The evidence suggests that some of the children need not have died. The Paediatric Death Review Committee of the College of Physicians and Surgeons, in its annual report for 1994, classified four of the twelve cases (without identifying which cases) as being possibly preventable with improved medical management. I believe that that number could be even higher.
>
> The evidence from these proceedings suggests that the deaths of Jessica Ulimaumi, Vinay Goyal, Marietess Capili, Jessie Maguire and Erin Petkau involved some form of mismanagement, surgical error or misadventure and were all at least possibly preventable or preventable. The operations on Daniel Terziski and Erica Bichel involved procedures that were probably outside the ability of the surgeon and the team to attempt and ought not to have been done in this province. The operation on Shalynn Piller was outside the permitted parameters applicable to the team at the time of the operation and also ought not to have been done in this province.
>
> The deaths of Gary Caribou, Alyssa Still and Ashton Feakes are still surrounded by more questions than answers. Only the death of Aric Baumann from a fatal and untreatable disease has been acceptably explained.

Professor Jan Davies analysed the Manitoba problem in terms of the following matrix (*see* Table 10.1).[89]

In the discussion at the end of this chapter, we shall compare the events in Bristol and Winnipeg, Manitoba and how they have affected policy.

**Table 10.1** Davies' analysis of the Manitoba problem[89]

| Components | 'Why?' Structure Latent conditions | 'How?' Process Active failures | 'What?' Outcome (multiple: O–1, O–2, O–3 …) |
|---|---|---|---|
| Patients | pre-operative characteristics | (1) referral for surgical treatment (2) discussion of options | (1) death (2) post-operative discussion |
| Personnel | individuals (1) training (2) experience | individuals (1) operative procedure(s) (2) charting (3) constant on-call (4) continued referrals | individuals (1) psychological (2) leave institution/ system (3) ↓ knowledge & skills |
| | OR team formation (1) culture (2) briefing (3) there was no 'team' | OR team maintenance (1) communication (2) conflict (3) debriefing (4) 'team' dysfunction | OR team conclusion (1) disbanding of 'team' |
| Environment | (1) Winnipeg • limited population (2) OR • size • temperature control • noise (3) ICU • separate PICU & NICU | (1) Winnipeg • limited number of procedures (2) OR • poor ergonomics • poor temperature control of room • impaired communication (3) ICU • division of no. of cases | (1) Winnipeg • limited expertise (2) OR • less than optimal performance • unstable thermoregulatory control of patients • ? death of Vinay Goyal (3) ICU • division of expertise |
| Equipment | (1) OR • lack of a drug • lack of TEE (2) ICU • lack of clamps | (1) OR • delay in administration • ↓ ability to perform intra-operative echo (2) ICU • impaired procedures | (1) OR • delay in coming off pump • ↓ knowledge of anatomy & function of heart (2) ICU • ECMO death |

**Table 10.1** Continued

| Components | 'Why?' Structure Latent conditions | 'How?' Process Active failures | 'What?' Outcome (multiple: O–1, O–2, O–3 …) |
|---|---|---|---|
| Organisation | (1) selection criteria & process | (1) no telephone follow-up of references | (1) lack of complete information about Dr Odim |
| | (2) policies & procedures | (2) inability to follow policies & procedures | (2) lack of information about organisation |
| | (3) staffing | (3) delay in autopsy results | (3) lack of information about patient outcomes |
| | (4) methods of evaluation | (4) ineffective evaluation • no rapid review of problems • reliance on M&M review • reliance on Standards Committee • reliance on Wiseman • Committee | (4) lack of information about the programme |
| | (5) management authority | (5) abdication of responsibility • no orientation • no follow-up of problems | (5) lack of information about the programme |
| | (6) restructuring | (6) impaired/ confused lines of communication | (6) lack of information about workplace and programme |
| | (7) culture | (7) poor or no flow of information | (7) lack of knowledge about the programme |
| Regulatory authorities: Department of Health | 'need for programme' despite low population | establishment of single surgeon programme | ? inappropriate programme |
| Manitoba Medical Association | inadequate $ for surgeon | loss of previous surgeon | programme dysfunction & dissolution |
| College of Physicians and Surgeons of Manitoba | Standards Committee | death review process | delay in acquiring information |

# Scandals in Australia

There has not been such a high-profile scandal in Australia as Bristol or Winnipeg, Manitoba. However, Professor Davies notes in her evidence to the Manitoba Pediatric Cardiac Surgery Inquest that:[89]

> From discussions with anaesthetists, I learned that there had been prob-
> lems with paediatric cardiac surgery in centres in Australia. In each centre,
> it was the anaesthetist(s) who had flagged the higher than expected
> morbidity and mortality. In one centre, for example, the anaesthetists
> withdrew services and no operations were performed for several months.
> An external audit was set up but the report of the reviewer was never
> made public. Several recommendations were made, including a move
> to the Children's Hospital. Currently, surgery is limited in complexity
> and the size/age of the child. Closed cases are done on small babies but
> bypass work is limited to older children with straightforward lesions.

This highlights one of the problems. Complex surgery is difficult and in spite of the impression created by the UK media, the children involved were very sick. Therefore we are dealing with the area of 'higher than expected morbidity and mortality'.

The issue becomes – at what point does this higher than expected result become an unacceptable problem? The lesson from Bristol is that the point comes earlier than some surgeons were prepared to admit.

Whilst the public profile of problems in the Australian system is not as high as the profile in the UK, the 1999 report of the National Expert Advisory Group commented on the need for better adverse incident reporting and recommended the establishment of the Australian Council for Safety and Quality in Healthcare. The Council was duly established in January 2000 and in July 2002 produced the major *Report into Obstetrics and Gynaecological Services at King Edward Memorial Hospital, 1990–2000.*[90]

The King Edward Memorial Hospital in Perth is Western Australia's only tertiary referral service for obstetrics and gynaecology. The Hospital receives and treats the most difficult and complex obstetric cases in Western Australia and operates 24 hours per day, seven days per week. The Hospital is the state's only major teaching hospital in obstetrics and gynaecology and is a centre for midwifery training and for postgraduate medical training.

It has 250 in-patient beds, 60 neonatal cots and intensive care services, and a range of out-patient services. Each year 5000 gynaecological operations are performed at the Hospital, approximately 5000 babies are born there and the Hospital's emergency centre has 8000–10 000 women presenting for gynaecological or obstetric treatment.

The inquiry report describes the situation at the hospital as follows:[90]

> In 1990 the Health Department of Western Australia commissioned the
> University of Western Australia's Professor of Obstetrics and Gynaecology
> to report on the state's future obstetric, gynaecological and neonatal ser-
> vice requirements. The report recommended changes at King Edward
> Memorial Hospital, including revision of obstetric staffing levels.

However, these recommendations were not implemented despite the Hospital medical and nursing clinicians repeatedly raising concerns about staffing levels with Hospital management throughout the 1990s. Nor was there any evidence that the Hospital management conveyed this information to the Health Department of Western Australia.

Concerned about important process and performance issues at the Hospital, the recently appointed Chief Executive wrote to the Metropolitan Health Service Board Chief Executive Officer in 1999 about the:

- lack of an overall clinical quality management system;
- problems identifying and rectifying clinical issues by senior management;
- inadequate systems to monitor and report adverse clinical incidents;
- absence of a proper and transparent system to deal with patient complaints and claims;
- shortage of qualified clinical specialists, particularly after hours;
- inadequate supervision of junior medical staff; and
- possibility of sub-standard patient care.

The Hospital's Chief Executive also outlined changes he had established to address these issues and recommended additional changes. After consultation with the Health Department's Chief Medical Officer, the Hospital's Chief Executive provided evidence of poor practice at the Hospital. As a result, the Metropolitan Health Service Board commissioned a review by an independent senior clinician to examine the issues. This review also raised concerns about significant clinical issues and recommended a more detailed investigation into the Hospital's obstetric and gynaecological services.

In consultation with the Commissioner of Health and the Minister, the Chief Medical Officer and the Metropolitan Health Service Board Chief Executive Officer commissioned the Child and Glover Review (2000). This two-week review identified significant system and performance issues. As a result, the Minister in consultation with the Premier agreed to establish the Douglas Inquiry under the Hospitals Act and the Public Sector Management Act.

Strong public debate arose from the high public profile given to the Hospital during this time and the issues raised about its future. Individual doctors and the Western Australian branch of the Australian Medical Association actively debated the issues, resulting in public criticism of the Child and Glover findings. The Douglas Inquiry's findings are consistent with those of the Child and Glover Review.

In the view that such problems arise from a combination of factors and inadequate systems, one of the problems facing the inquiry was the state of clinical records:[90]

> Of all cases reviewed, the care plan was inadequate or non-existent in 20 per cent of cases and important documentation was inadequate in 35 per cent of cases and missing in 15 per cent of cases.

The quality and completeness of documentation varied across the Hospital. Outcomes of discussions with senior staff were rarely noted. In most cases it was impossible to determine the extent of a consultant's involvement in decisions about care. Senior medical staff provided some of the worst examples of poor record keeping and it was rare for a consultant to document a plan or record care. Most entries were illegible and most signatures were indecipherable. File notes were disjointed, incomplete and disorganised. Pre-operative assessment was usually absent and many notes were sketchy and difficult to understand. Private physicians generally failed to record antenatal care as a reference for the Hospital clinicians.

There were clear consequences of this for clinical care, leading to a high rate of clinical errors:

Of the 372 high-risk obstetric cases reviewed, errors were common, and the most frequent were 'failure to recognise a serious and unstable condition' and 'inappropriate omissions'. Of the cases reviewed:

- one or more clinical errors occurred in 47 per cent of cases;
- 50 per cent of these were very serious;
- junior residents made errors in 76 per cent of high-risk cases;
- junior registrars made errors in 65 per cent of high-risk cases;
- midwives made errors in 60 per cent of high-risk cases;
- levels 5 and 6 registrars made errors in 34 per cent of high-risk cases; and
- consultants made errors in 28 per cent of high-risk cases.

The healthcare professionals recognised the failings in the system. For example, midwives established their own procedures to report adverse events in the form of a paper-based register. This unofficial and incomplete record identified 47 incidents for the period July 1998 to June 2000. The inquiry reviewed 30 of these in detail, and 19 involved moderately unsafe or very unsafe practices. Of the 605 clinical files reviewed, 71 cases with moderately unsafe or very unsafe practices occurred in the Obstetrics Clinical Care Unit from July 1998 to June 2000. Of these, only 19 were recorded in the register. Staff frequently used email to report obstetric incidents.

Of the 605 cases reviewed, eight reportable deaths were found and sent by the inquiry to the Coroner. Of these, the care of the woman and baby was graded as very unsafe in six cases and as moderately unsafe in one case. The Coroner advised that none of these deaths had been reported previously.

Staff repeatedly raised serious concerns about management and clinical issues with their clinical director and with non-clinical administrators. However these matters remained unresolved, often being referred to internal hospital committees, who did nothing in response.

Over a long period of years, many problems remained unresolved:

- non-existent or sub-standard care planning and coordination
- poor management of high-risk cases and medical emergencies

- lack of supervision of junior medical staff
- inadequate staff skills profile in the adult special care unit
- sub-standard documentation adversely affecting care continuity
- non-existent systems for identifying, reviewing and responding to adverse events.

The perceptions of many women and their families were that they received little or no information about their treatment options, risks or errors of care. During the review period, women and their families reported:

- inadequate information about their treatment and little or no involvement in decisions about care
- inadequate or no information about things that went wrong and what was being done about the situation
- poor treatment and disrespect when making a complaint
- lack of support when they experienced poor outcomes or adverse events
- poor or no communication from hospital staff during potential medical negligence case reviews.

The inquiry identified the following key findings:

- The lack of safety and quality systems at state, board and hospital level was evidenced by ineffective accreditation and credentialling systems, inadequate incident reporting systems, poorly performing statutory mortality reporting and investigation systems, and non-existent inter-hospital comparative data analysis. At hospital level, the inquiry found many examples of exemplary care and significant effort on the part of individuals to overcome long-standing clinical and management problems. However, the inquiry also found significant leadership, management and clinical performance problems, including a culture of blame, unsupportive of open disclosure of errors and adverse events;
- lack of clarification of senior staff responsibilities and accountability;
- non-existent 'safety nets' or systems to effectively monitor performance and respond to performance issues;
- ineffective or non-existent systems to ensure staff had the right credentials, training, support and performance management to meet the demands and skill requirements of their roles and responsibilities;
- failure to meet the emotional needs of many women and their families, excluding them from decisions about care or failing to give them honest, complete and timely information when things went wrong; and
- failure to address serious and ongoing management and clinical problems that resulted in serious adverse events and poor outcomes for women and their families.

The most staggering conclusions are the length of time over which the problems persisted, and the difficulty in establishing the actual impact of the problems on patient outcomes due to the period elapsed and the poor quality of record keeping.

# What are the common factors and lessons from these incidents?

The superficial similarities between Bristol and Winnipeg are striking. Many of the lessons to be learned apply in both cases.

The first area of common concern is communication both pre- and post-operatively. Pre-operatively, in both situations, there were documented cases where the risk reported to parents was considerably less than the actual risk:[91]

> A major issue in the Bristol case has been the nature of the information given to the parents. The estimates of risk of death were substantially less than the true risk of surgery in that unit. There may be a place for giving an optimistic outlook to a patient judged to have no choice but to undergo high-risk emergency surgery to save life, but the circumstances where that approach is justified are limited. There was no justification for a rosy glow in this case, where the operations were elective, could be performed elsewhere and the difference between success and failure was potentially many years of life. It appears to be self-evident that parents have a right to know the truth from both referring cardiologist and the surgeon.
>
> Why are doctors ever economical with it? Is truth thought to contaminate the trust in a relationship? A frank presentation of the risks and benefits to the family should include sympathy and compassion, but this should not supplant frankness.

In the Winnipeg case, the inquest also heard that parents were not informed of true risks:[89]

> No one told Charlotte Caribou that the surgeon had never before performed this type of surgery on this type of patient without supervision. She was unaware of the fact that the surgical team had performed only a very few simple operations together. Additionally, she was never told that her son's chest condition placed him at increased risk for the procedure he was undergoing.

Post-operatively, in both Bristol and Winnipeg, the parents heard of major problems from the media, greatly exacerbating their distress and anger.

In both cases, the surgeons were learning new techniques, with the complicating factor that neither was experienced in paediatric surgery. One UK paediatrician commented to me that prior to Bristol, some surgeons regarded paediatric surgery as 'practice for adult surgery'. In neither case did the institution have appropriate systems for mentoring new staff, or adequate data to monitor their performance.

The final major similarity is in the role of 'whistle blowers' in making matters public. In Bristol, the situation was made public by a whistle blower. In Winnipeg, Manitoba there was no whistle blower, but the threat of revelation was a factor:[89]

> The issue of whistle blowing was raised with the inquest as something that required redress in Manitoba's medical care system. There does appear to be merit to that view. In this case, none of the persons involved actually went outside the processes available to address the concerns

they had. While those with concerns appear to have spoken with all those in positions of authority who they could identify, none of their actions came close to involving people who were outside the very institution that had a responsibility to do something about those concerns. However, the concern that Youngson had about going to speak to authorities outside the hospital and the personal and professional risk she ran on doing so, point to the need for change in this area. Chapter ten contains recommendations for changes to protect whistle blowers.

In both cases their concerns were raised internally first, but ignored or overruled.

The biggest difference between the situations was the speed of reaction. The problems in Winnipeg were recognised much more quickly than those in Bristol; attempts were made to correct them and when this failed, surgery was halted. Ultimately, this led to fewer deaths as a consequence.

In the Australian case, the inquiry team noted the following similarities to Bristol:

- serious problems being identified by whistle blowers rather than being identified and addressed or prevented through rigorous and routine safety and quality monitoring systems
- both cases called for changes to encourage transparency and monitoring in an open fashion
- failure at government, board and management level to establish a culture of inquiry and open disclosure, and to introduce systems to monitor and improve the safety and quality of healthcare.

The lessons highlighted also are strikingly similar:[90]

- To assure safe, quality care, governments, boards, healthcare leaders and managers must create an open and transparent culture, where people willingly discuss and address errors and systems problems.
- Effective organisations have people at all levels doing the right thing. Organisational structures, regardless of their intent or design, can only be effective if people know and aim to meet their responsibilities and are held accountable for their actions.
- Effective leaders and managers ensure that their organisation has systems that effectively monitor the key aspects of its performance, and ensure timely and appropriate responses to performance issues.
- To do a good job, people need the right credentials, training, support, performance management and development consistent with the demands and skills requirements of their roles and responsibilities.
- A caring, concerned healthcare service recognises the importance of involving patients and their families in care, provides information about care options, involves them in decisions about care and advises them openly and honestly when things go wrong.

Many of these issues also applied in the Winnipeg case. In all three cases, a common theme was the poor treatment of patients and their carers. In Winnipeg and Perth, Western Australia, a further common theme was the failure to act upon internal reviews which were later vindicated by external scrutiny.

# Have they influenced policy and practice?

There is little doubt that Bristol, and to a lesser extent Alder Hey and Shipman, have left NHS policy 'all changed, changed utterly'.[85]

There has been a raft of policy initiatives in response to the recommendations of the Bristol inquiry.[92] In this report, the Government summarised its response in a series of objectives:

> In responding to the challenge set by the Kennedy Report, the key tasks which lie ahead of us are to:
>
> - put patients at the centre of the NHS;
> - improve children's healthcare services;
> - set, inspect and monitor the standards of care (the roles of CHI, NICE and NPSA);
> - ensure the safety of care;
> - develop a health service which is well led and managed;
> - improve the regulation, education and training of healthcare professionals;
> - improve the quality, reliability and range of information which supports decision making and strengthen the monitoring of performance; and
> - involve patients and the public in healthcare.
>
> 12 We are committed to changing attitudes in the way care is delivered. We want to develop a culture of openness, honesty and trust to ensure that patients have the information they need to make informed choices and to enable patients to become equal partners with healthcare professionals in making decisions about treatment and care.
>
> 13 Our programme of reform will include:
> - more information provided to patients on how local health services compare with others and greater choice for patients over where they are treated;
> - a consent process which engages patients fully in decisions about their care;
> - an Expert Patient Programme to support the development of partnerships between clinicians and patients from late 2001;
> - from April 2003, a National Knowledge Service for the NHS to support the delivery of high-quality information for patients and staff;
> - the establishment of Patient Advice and Liaison Services (PALS) within every trust from April 2002 to assist patients in managing and accessing information;
> - by the summer of 2002, guidelines about sharing information with patients and parents of young children;
> - a review of bereavement services;
> - publication of a Code of Practice on communicating with families about post-mortems in January 2002; and
> - a reformed NHS complaints procedure by December 2002.
>
> (Executive summary, Government's response to
> the Kennedy Report[92])

One of the major impacts of the UK scandals has been the erosion of confidence in doctors as a profession. In May 2002, the Government published a consultation document on reforming the General Medical Council, the body responsible for 'policing' the medical profession.[93] Central to the proposals are the requirements for doctors to demonstrate their continuing competence to practise, known as 'revalidation'.

Nurses asked about this point to the fact that their profession has had this system for years. The more cynical of them comment that it represents a diminution in the doctor's privileged position in the healthcare team and that this is an appropriate response to the problems at Bristol and Winnipeg.

Most of these responses relate to the reorganisation of the professionals and their systems. These are designed to identify and prevent catastrophic failure such as occurred in Bristol and Winnipeg.

The impact on the routine care of patients will be less immediate and will depend upon the measures having the desired effect and changes in culture. You cannot legislate to change the doctor–patient relationship: procedures only facilitate changes in culture.

A danger is that the new systems will encourage defensive behaviours. For example, increased monitoring may discourage doctors from carrying out high-risk operations.

On a more mundane level, one of the UK Government's responses to Bristol has been the introduction of many more guidelines and standards for doctors. These are superficially attractive and 'evidence based'. However, at best, the evidence is based upon a population average. Doctors faced with an individual patient with specific needs may be strongly discouraged from using their own judgement to take account of these needs by a defensive and litigious culture.

In Canada, the impact of the Winnipeg deaths has been less than that of Bristol in the UK. The most obvious reason is the provincial nature of Canada and the consequent regulatory framework:[94]

> Recommendations from the Bristol Inquiry have been noted throughout the United Kingdom, while those from Winnipeg seem not to have had much direct effect outside the province. Healthcare regulation is conducted at different levels in these two jurisdictions: it is 'national' for Bristol and 'provincial' for Winnipeg. Despite the fact that the Canada Health Act assures universality and portability, provincial borders can – and do – act as barriers to the identification, dissemination, access and use of information and recommendations from such inquiries.
>
> (Professor Jan Davies, *Canadian Medical Association Journal* editorial)

Other Canadian commentators noted that the lesser impact was due to the relative isolation of Winnipeg:

> If it had happened in Toronto then it would have had a much bigger impact, but people outside of Manitoba just said 'well that's Winnipeg for you'.
>
> (Former Winnipeg resident now living in Toronto)

Another commented on the greater power of the doctors' associations in Canada to resist change in regulation.

The author's experience in Australia was that there was remarkably little concern over issues like Bristol, in spite of the author's work coinciding with the inquiry into King Edward Hospital and the original report having been in the public domain since 2000. Reasons for this may be:

- the geographical remoteness of Perth from the eastern coast of Australia where the research was based
- the attitude identified above in relation to Winnipeg that it occurred in some where regarded as backward compared to the major centres
- the fact that many of the problems related to adults, whose care is less emotive than children.

In reality, many of the changes identified in the aftermath of Bristol were highlighted in Australia through initiatives such as the *Final Report to Health Ministers* from the National Expert Advisory Group on Safety and Quality in Australian Healthcare.[95]

In spite of all the noise and media attention, it is questionable how much these sad cases have impacted upon practice. In the UK, where there has been the most public impact, the vast range of NHS policy initiatives arising from Bristol have been subsumed within an even greater number of modernising initiatives.

The scandals have provided the Government with ammunition to push through the reforms that they would wish to pursue anyway. The biggest impact has been upon doctors' status and the change in culture which now means that it is acceptable to ask questions about a doctor's clinical practice. Even so, many patients would agree with the sentiments of one midwife who, expressing a view as a patient, said:

> Doctors? Arrogant and overpaid as a profession, but mine's a saint.
>
> (UK midwife)

In Canada and Australia, there seems to be a view that they simply represent local difficulties rather than systemic weaknesses. Perhaps the most telling quotes are from the report into the King Edward Hospital:[90]

> There is no way of knowing how the Hospital's performance compares overall with other Australian hospitals.

and from Professor Davies' *CMAJ* editorial:[94]

> If we do not, then the stories in Bristol and Winnipeg are 'bound to be retold elsewhere'.*

---

*This is a reference to a *Lancet* **351** editorial, 'First lessons from the Bristol case'. You can access the whole editorial on-line by going through a free registration process. The *Lancet* website is accessible from the website accompanying this book.

# CHAPTER 11

# Driver 3: ideology

## How ideology has driven policy in the UK

Healthcare is amongst the highest priorities for any Government. Therefore, it follows that healthcare is highly politicised and driven by ideology as much as evidence and effectiveness.

The reforms of the NHS under Mrs Thatcher from 1986 onwards were clearly driven by a set of political beliefs:

- free market economics
- competition as a mechanism for improving quality
- patient choice.

These were enshrined in the reforms of the day centred upon the 'internal market', which divided the NHS into purchasers and providers of healthcare. One of the most touted of these reforms was the introduction of GP fund-holding. I reviewed fund-holding in 1998. The conclusion to that paper was:[96]

> Fund-holding in the UK has a bleak future. This is not because primarily of any of the evidence provided in this paper, but because of the ideological allegiances of the major political parties in the UK. If the previous Conservative Government had been re-elected, then fund-holding would now be being further expanded. Since the Labour Government was elected in May 1997, fund-holding has been suspended and is effectively to be phased out in favour of GP commissioning, where groups of GPs combine to obtain services from hospitals. This emphasises the new ethos of cooperation rather than competition, a key feature of the NHS since 1989.
>
> The new Government claim to have saved £20m in administrative costs by rejecting all current applications for fund-holding.
>
> This ideological decision making is not necessarily helpful. The total fund-holding pilots had not completed their first year of operation let alone been evaluated when it was announced that it was a success and the scheme was to be expanded.

The conclusion has been broadly vindicated by events since. The point may be illustrated further from the 1997 *New NHS* White Paper:[15]

> This White Paper marks a turning point for the NHS. It replaces the internal market with integrated care. We are saving £1 billion of red

tape and putting that money into front-line patient care. For the first time the need to ensure that high-quality care is spread throughout the service will be taken seriously. National standards of care will be guaranteed. There will be easier and swifter access to the NHS when you need it. Our approach combines efficiency and quality with a belief in fairness and partnership.

(Tony Blair, Prime Minister, Foreword)

There were problems with the internal market:

- The market depends upon spare capacity in the system to make it work. The NHS was characterised by a lack of capacity rather than a surplus.
- Many patients and GPs had no choice over their provider in practice due to geographical constraints.
- It was deemed to be unfair and inequitable, especially between fund-holding and non-fund-holding practices.
- Transactions costs were often prohibitively expensive, and hospitals had no effective costing mechanisms in place.
- Providers who got their sums wrong could simply claw back the money at the end of the financial year from purchasers.
- If this didn't work, no hospital would ever be allowed to go bust, so they would be bailed out anyway.

However, the commitment to replace the internal market with integrated care has not yet happened five years on.

The same ideological need to turn things on their head is seen a year later in the information strategy document *Information for Health*:[97]

Up to now the use of IT in the NHS has not been a success story. Far from it. Lots of money has been wasted. Some important data have not been collected and used. Other data have been collected but not used. There has been too much emphasis on financial data to support an internal market at the expense of IT systems which could directly benefit patients. As a result, clinicians working in the NHS came to see data collection not as a help but as a hindrance to their work.

(Foreword)

However, this Government has adopted a more pragmatic approach to implementation in recent years. *Realpolitik* required the Government to stick to the previous administration's spending limits in their first administration. There seems to be little doubt that in spite of this, local NHS trusts were allowed to run up large overspends or deficits in order to attempt to bring down waiting times.

Now that new funds are being released, the first call on additional funds is often to pay overspends from previous years. More significant is the Government's enthusiastic adoption of the Private Finance Initiative. This was an initiative of the previous administration, and its basis in the private sector place sets it clearly at ideological odds with the traditional stance of Labour Governments. This has led to opposition from traditional allies such as the trade unions.

More significant is the announcement in the 2002 *NHS Annual Report*:[98]

> Other measures in the pipeline will give the NHS the freedom to improve
> local services to patients. We will extend the Private Finance Initiative,
> encourage joint ventures with the private and voluntary sectors, maxi-
> mise the NHS use of spare private sector hospital capacity and bring
> overseas clinical teams into the country to work for the NHS. Soon the
> first NHS foundation hospitals will be identified, with new freedoms
> to raise standards of care further.
>
> (Secretary of State for Health)

These foundation hospitals will have more freedom to raise money by borrowing,
and to set local conditions of pay and service. They represent a system which is a
logical extension of the internal market that operated between 1992 and 1997, but
which takes the concept further than the previous administration.

All the same arguments that were levelled against the internal market can be
levelled against this new wave of 'foundation hospitals'.

Lest anyone should feel that this Government has completely embraced pragmatism and stopped behaving like a Government, the reference to local services
both in the foundation hospitals and in the newly established primary care trusts
is matched by the most rigorous set of national standards and control mechanisms ever seen, justified in the name of patient safety and as a response to Bristol
and other problems:[74]

> Patients should have fair access and high standards of care wherever
> they live. So at national level the Department of Health will, with the
> help of leading clinicians, managers and staff, set national standards in
> the priority areas. These standards will take three forms:
>
> - *National standards for key conditions and diseases through National Service
>   Frameworks (NSFs)*. NSFs have already been produced covering
>   mental health and coronary heart disease and in the autumn will be
>   followed by the country's first ever comprehensive National Cancer
>   Plan. An NSF for older people's services will be published in Autumn
>   2000 and for diabetes next year. These five service frameworks between
>   them cover around half of total NHS spending. Further NSFs will be
>   developed on a rolling basis over the period of the Plan.
> - *Clear guidance on the best treatments and interventions from the National
>   Institute for Clinical Excellence (NICE)*. Its work is helping to ensure a
>   faster, more uniform uptake of treatments which work best for patients.
>   This year the National Institute for Clinical Excellence is due to under-
>   take 23 appraisals and to issue ten sets of guidelines. As part of
>   *The NHS Plan* we will increase the work programme of the National
>   Institute for Clinical Excellence. It will carry out 50% more appraisals
>   and produce 50% more guidelines. To enable it to carry out this extra
>   work we will increase the National Institute for Clinical Excellence
>   budget by £2 million.
> - *A limited number of ambitious but achievable national targets*. They will
>   include shorter waiting times, the quality of care and facilities for

people while they are in hospital, new services to help people remain independent and efficiency.

This Government arrived with a pure ideological position, at least in its presentation. However, it has gradually revealed a more pragmatic agenda. The only major ideological factor which distinguishes it from the previous administration is overall spending which is considerably higher and rising.

# How ideology has driven policy in Canada

Canada is unique in that the central level of government plays a very small direct role in the delivery of healthcare. Under the Canadian Constitution, healthcare is a matter of provincial/territorial jurisdiction except in the case of some groups of people, the most important being the First Nations and the Inuit. Historically, the Federal Government, at a time when its share of overall healthcare spending was more important than it is now, had a controlling influence on the development of the Canadian healthcare delivery system which culminated in the Canada Health Act.

The ideology that drives healthcare in Canada is unique and is based not on traditional political ideologies, but rather defined by the two foundations of the Canadian healthcare systems:

- the Federal/Provincial split
- the Canada Health Act.

The influence of the Federal/Provincial split was highlighted by a number of analysts in their evidence to the Romanow Commission. Carolyn Hughes Tuohy pointed to three strategies for enacting and implementing healthcare reform:[99]

> A big bang approach to healthcare reform is very politically risky and it is rare that any Government will take that chance. It requires a confluence or convergence of political developments that is very rare. You must be able to consolidate political authority on a fairly massive scale and you must have the political will to take the risk. To the extent that you consolidate authority, you also consolidate accountability, which then makes it more difficult to shift the blame to someone else.
>
> We have seen big bang reforms on rare occasions. We saw it in Britain after the Second World War with the establishment of the NHS. We saw it in the 1980s in Britain with the Thatcher Government in its third successive majority mandate. These are rare events.
>
> Blueprint-type reforms are more likely in coalition circumstances where bipartisan compromise is necessary. I have not mentioned certain US states where we also saw blueprint approaches because of the need for bipartisan compromise – with a similar result as that in the Netherlands. Things tended to stall or get rolled back as the complexion of the political coalition changed over time.
>
> In Australia and Canada we have seen incremental reforms where Federal-Provincial consensus cannot be mobilized for something broader. That, also, is a result of factors in the broad political arena and not in the healthcare arena itself.

Overall, proposals for a 'big bang' overhaul of Canada's healthcare system would be difficult. Nonetheless, major changes are needed if the hopes and aspirations of Canadians are to be met. A former health minister in Québec, in evidence to the same Committee, pointed out the dangers of solutions based upon ideology in systems where the political flavour of the Government may change rapidly:[100]

> It appears that there are many instances of practical solutions being attempted [in Western Europe]. However, those systems are closely related with the political lives of their respective country, which means that the attempts are fragile. These experiments are not sustained, even when successful.
>
> I would not condemn any system for attempting new solutions and changing its mind when new solutions are not effective. However, this has not been the case. The closeness of the system to the political life of the country means that ideological reasons are the cause of the system's failure.
>
> We [in Canada] share that habit to some extent. It should alert us to the danger of a public system that is held hostage by the vagaries of political life. When the healthcare system is tied to the political system it fails to sustain a pragmatic, managerial approach to problem solving.
> (Claude Forget, in Evidence to the Romanow Commission)

In practice, in Canada, the Canada Health Act has achieved a consensus around it which goes beyond political allegiance, and therefore has a stronger ideological status than any political view on this issue.

However, as with all ideologies, the pure ideology does not represent the reality. Whilst ideologically a public system, Canada has 30% private contribution to total healthcare costs, comparable with Australia and considerably more than the UK, whether measured as a percentage or as an absolute figure per capita.

The Romanow report has largely maintained the *status quo*, in spite of the author's claim to the contrary:[101]

> I cannot say often enough that the *status quo* IS NOT AN OPTION!

The report specifically reaffirms the fundamental principles of the Canada Health Act and adds accountability. It seeks to extend the scope of Medicare, and specifically seeks to reduce private provision in areas of direct care to patients. Even the areas where it seeks reform it does so by asserting the sanctity of the principles of the Act:[60]

> Drugs, once a small portion of total health costs, are now escalating and among the highest costs in the system. The expense associated with some drug therapies or of providing extended home care for a seriously ill family member can be financially devastating. It can bankrupt a family. This is incompatible with the philosophy and values upon which Medicare was built. It must be changed. I am therefore recommending that home care be recognized as a publicly insured service under Medicare and that, as a priority, new funds be invested to establish a national platform for home care services.

> I am also recommending the creation of a national drug strategy, including a catastrophic drug insurance program to protect Canadian families.
>
> (p.xvii)

The report retains the values of the Canada Health Act, and seeks to modernise them in the light of changes to society and the healthcare system since the original Act. The report affirms the view of the McGill Medical Faculty:[60]

> Medicare has as much iconic force here as the Constitution does in the USA.
>
> (p.47)

The report is perhaps surprisingly limited in its findings on waiting times and its reforms to address them. It acknowledges three areas for concern:[60]

- access to advanced diagnostic technologies such as magnetic resonance imaging (MRI) and computed tomography (CT) scanners;
- access to specialists (though this varies greatly between specialties, between provinces and even within provinces); and
- access to some surgical procedures (e.g. hip and knee replacements) that may not be life-saving but would improve the patient's quality of life.

> (pp.139–40)

But it argues that the most effective intervention is to increase diagnostic testing to remove a bottleneck in the system. It seems possible that this will simply create demand that cannot be satisfied elsewhere in the system. This is in spite of the report quoting patient experiences that seem very familiar to UK audiences:[60]

> I am one of that great cadre called 'elective' patients. We are not seen as emergencies.... I have recently had a hip replacement; I was waiting for that replacement for almost two years.... The word 'elective' is offensive; it isn't as though we're going to the store to buy some shrimp versus some liver: we have no choice about using the healthcare system.
>
> I go to Emergency when I am sick; there are no other choices. Waiting to see a specialist is a long-term wait, usually about 6–12 months.
>
> (Patient submissions to the Romanow Commission, pp.138–9)

# How ideology has driven policy in Australia

Australia has the most overtly ideological approach to healthcare. The right-wing Howard administration has constantly encouraged more and more private sector in all aspects of healthcare:

- huge incentives to take out private insurance for individuals
- increased ownership of general practices by commercial organisations
- vertical integration by commercial organisations.

The Government remains committed to private provision of healthcare:[102]

> According to the figures released by the Private Health Administration
> Council (PHIAC), the proportion of the population covered by private
> insurance in the September quarter was 44%, although the number of
> people covered increased by 4268 to 8 709 000.
>     Senator Patterson said: 'This is an excellent result and demonstrates,
> yet again, the success of the Howard Government's determination to
> restore the balance to our healthcare system.'
>     'Only recently, we saw that in 2000–2001, for the very first time in the
> history of Medicare, the number of public hospital admissions fell, by
> almost 5000. At the same time, the number of private hospital admissions
> grew by a massive 245 000. Importantly, these figures do not include
> the real impact of Lifetime Health Cover.'
>     'Clearly, we have restored the balance to our healthcare system and
> taken pressure off Medicare and the public hospital system.'

Whilst this may meet the ideological goal of increasing the uptake of private
healthcare, it has only a marginal effect on the waiting lists.

In 2001–02, the Government's own data showed a marginal fall in the waiting
list (*see* Table 11.1).

However, the number treated as elective surgery cases is about 12% less than
the numbers added to the waiting list.

The final figure for removals from the waiting list includes over 30 000 who
were removed for reasons that were not recorded, another 36 000 for whom
surgery was not required or declined, nearly 8000 who died and nearly 3000 who
were admitted as emergencies.

This is against a background of falling private expenditure on healthcare and
increasing public expenditure.

The point has been made elsewhere that there is very little evidence that private
provision can be managed as cost-effectively as public sector operation. In spite of
all of this, my conversations with Australians were not marked by the same anxiety
amongst patients or professionals about access to care as those in the UK and
Canada. Australians generally believe that their system gives them choice and access
to services, in a way that British people don't and Canadians doubt.

From a political perspective, this may be regarded as a successful outcome and
the level of expenditure, currently broadly on a par with Canada in terms of both
total expenditure and its public/private split, may be seen as an acceptable price to
pay.

# Conclusions

There can be no doubt that politics and ideology are major drivers in the three systems under scrutiny. In practice, however, the direction is not obvious or simple.

In Australia, we have the clearest link with political ideology. The Government
trumpets the adoption of private healthcare as an end in itself. This position is not
unlike the position of the Thatcher Government in the UK, which whilst recognising
that a direct and overt move to private healthcare would be politically undesirable,

**Table 11.1** Waiting list summary data, 2001–02[103]

| | NSW | Vic | Qld | WA | SA | Tas | ACT | NT | Total |
|---|---|---|---|---|---|---|---|---|---|
| **Additions** | **218 477** | **129 156** | **123 854** | **44 251** | **38 109** | **15 361** | **7264** | **7630** | **584 102** |
| **Removals** | | | | | | | | | |
| Admitted as an elective patient | 192 867 | 110 388 | 104 688 | 39 438 | 35 562 | 12 995 | 6836 | 5516 | 508 290 |
| Admitted as an emergency admission | 1578 | 628 | n.a. | 292 | 187 | n.a. | 3 | 7 | 2695 |
| Could not be contacted/died | 3670 | 1740 | n.a. | 790 | 442 | 731 | 244 | n.a. | 7617 |
| Treated elsewhere | 8196 | 4005 | n.a. | 1283 | 916 | 584 | 314 | n.a. | 15 298 |
| Surgery not required or declined | 14 890 | 9714 | n.a. | 6816 | 1850 | 1085 | 1567 | n.a. | 35 922 |
| Not reported | .. | 3842 | 18 916 | 1218 | 1076 | .. | 1558 | 3820 | 30 430 |
| **Total removals** | **221 201** | **130 317** | **123 604** | **49 837** | **40 033** | **15 395** | **10 522** | **9343** | **600 252** |

measured the success of their reforms in measures such as the uptake of GP fund-holding rather than its impact upon health outcomes.

The current UK Government started by adopting a largely ideological position, e.g. in its abandonment of fund-holding, but in practice has adopted a much more pragmatic approach and increasingly is adopting measures such as the Private Finance Initiative and foundation hospitals that are ideologically at odds with their traditional position.

Canada represents a different situation. The Provincial/Federal split is much stronger than its corresponding relationship in Australia between Commonwealth and States. This, together with the reverence in which the Canada Health Act is held, means that ideological battles tend to form around defending the Act (or not) rather than traditional political lines.

# CHAPTER 12

# So what is a good healthcare system?

## The answer

By now you will have read 11 chapters and for the dedicated, over 100 additional sources of information. (If you skipped the previous 11 chapters, hoping just to find the answer, shame on you!) You have journeyed from the plains of Canada to the surfing beaches of Western Australia. You may feel justified in seeking a simple answer to the question. The bad news is that there isn't one.

As stated in Chapter 3, it all depends upon where you are looking at it from. One of the over-riding impressions, having carried out the research necessary to write this book, is that decision makers, whether in Government or management locally, make decisions on the basis of the population as a whole.

The reality of healthcare is that it represents a massive number of individual interactions between people, that people respond to as individuals. Whilst it may be necessary for decision makers to look at things from the macro level, losing sight of the micro level will result in bad decisions. Consider, for example, the parents in Bristol and Winnipeg. All the evidence points to the fact that these bad decisions were the result of systems failures and responses needed to be systematic. However, one of the major turning points in both cases was the point where the hospitals went public with the information that there were significant problems. Nearly all the parents heard about the problems from the media, making a nightmare experience even worse.

What is striking is how far removed much of the debate about policy is to the needs of the individual patients. The book started with three individuals. We left them at the end of Chapter 2 and we have not been near them since. To illustrate how this works, the UK Government talks in terms of a 'postcode lottery' about access to care. Either we have consistency across the system or we have a system able to respond to local need.

In reality, what the patients want is access to care when they need it and whether or not their counterparts in another part of the country are able to access care more quickly is of little interest at that time. On the other hand, some of the attributes of a good healthcare system are only seen in their absence. For example, a good healthcare system would provide you with access to care when you need it. A better system would prevent you from having that need if possible, by keeping you healthy.

# The reality

I suggest that Andrew, Anna, Daphne and Harold want three fundamental things from the healthcare system:

- They want it to keep them healthy if possible.
- Where this is not possible, they want it to make them better if possible.
- They want it to do this at the minimum cost consistent with these goals.

However, they then have a whole set of expectations that may be characterised as the required level of service. If the three primary requirements are what we require a system to do, then the levels of service determine how well we expect them to be done.

It is not acceptable for a modern healthcare system to merely keep people alive; it is expected to maintain a quality of life, both in terms of the impact on the patients' lives themselves and the way that care is provided. However, it should never be forgotten that the basic responsibility of the healthcare system is to deliver the basics. There are large parts of the world where basic provision as defined in Western countries is an unrealisable dream. Even in the countries examined in this book, the parents from Bristol and Winnipeg or the friends and relatives of Dr Shipman's victims would argue that *in extremis*, basic care is the priority.

One of the key challenges is to provide better service that does not conflict with the basic care. Consider, for example, a pregnancy such as Daphne's. For the vast majority of mothers and babies whose deliveries go without a need for major medical intervention, a home delivery is a safe option which protects the baby from the risk of infection in a hospital situation and may be more relaxing for the mother. However, for those mothers with serious complications, hospital is clearly safer. The challenge is to provide the best care on an individual basis. Effective risk management is required to prevent the small minority of cases that need hospitalisation from dominating the majority of cases.

# How well are the systems providing the basics?

The two simplest, if not best, indicators of basic performance in terms of health and cost may be considered as life expectancy at birth and cost measured relative to national wealth, characterised as % GDP.

Figure 12.1 illustrates performance in these terms. The graph is based upon 1999 data, the latest available for most OECD countries at the time of writing. The life expectancy figure at birth is based upon females as they interact more often with the healthcare system and therefore are more likely to be influenced by it. The best performance is at the top left-hand corner of the graph.

Of the countries we have considered, only Australia gets into the top left-hand quadrant. The UK narrowly misses out on life expectancy grounds, and Canada misses out on cost grounds. The USA, however, spends far more and achieves markedly less. In contrast, Japan achieves considerably more for less expenditure.

The data confirm the view that the UK is obtaining good results for the money it is spending, Canada better results by spending more and Australia slightly better results than Canada for slightly less money.

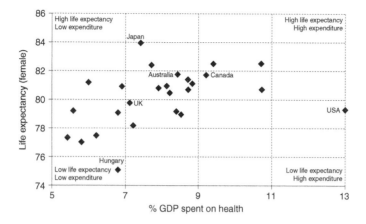

**Figure 12.1**   Life expectancy relative to expenditure.[44]

However, where the UK is often criticised is not in those areas but rather around non-life-threatening aspects, e.g. access to care for elective surgery.

# How well would the different systems meet the individual expectations and needs?

In order to consider other issues, we shall consider how well the systems that we have looked at would meet the needs and expectations of our four patients (*see* Table 12.1).

# What does our analysis tell us about the general characteristics of a good healthcare system?

In spite of the complexity of the issues, there are some overall conclusions which do seem to be supported by the evidence:

- *Private provision costs more.* In all three systems there does seem to be evidence that private provision adds to overall healthcare costs. In spite of this, all three systems are currently boosting private expenditure at present:
  - the UK is using its Private Finance Initiative to fund capital expansion
  - Canada is using its exclusion of drug costs and home care costs from the Canada Health Act to contain total public expenditure on health
  - Australia is blatantly providing massive and expensive tax incentives to its citizens to take out private insurance.
- *An increased role for primary care may improve healthcare in a cost-effective way.* In the late 1980s, the UK Conservative Government realised that health promotion and prevention in primary care was cheaper than increasing capacity in secondary

**Table 12.1** Our patients in the different national systems

| Patient | Australia | Canada | UK |
|---|---|---|---|
| Andrew | The Australian primary care system provides Andrew with the option of visiting a doctor near his office. He can afford to pay any fees required, so the system appears to meet his needs well. | Again Andrew would benefit from the freedom to use primary care facilities near his work. Any physician would be happy to provide a whole range of services in the light of the fee-for-service remuneration. | In the UK, Andrew will be targeted by his registered GP and encouraged to visit for a check-up. However, as stated earlier, a man of Andrew's age is unlikely to take up the offer unless he perceives he is ill. Also his registered GP will be near his home and it will not be convenient for Andrew to visit the surgery at the appointed time. |
| Anna | The Australian primary care system provides Anna with a great deal of choice over where she seeks advice. She can walk in off the street for advice from a GP who has never met her and this may be an attractive option. On the other hand, her choice may be restricted by the need to pay consultation charges in many practices. Should she opt for a programme of contraception based around the Pill, there is likely to be less systematic follow-up than in the UK due to the patient registration system in the UK. | The Canadian primary care system also provides Anna with a great deal of choice over where she seeks advice. She can walk in off the street for advice from a GP who has never met her and this may be an attractive option. Additionally, the absence of consultation fees may also encourage her. On the other hand, the doctor-centred system may prove something of a barrier. Should she opt for a programme of contraception based around the Pill, there is likely to be less systematic follow-up than in the UK due the patient registration system in the UK. On the other hand, the doctor-centred system may prove something of a barrier. | Anna may perceive a number of barriers in the UK system. She is registered with the practice that she has attended since birth, and where her parents are registered. She may not be aware that she can visit another GP in the same practice or even feel that this is still too close. Some UK GPs have also expressed concern that the growth of electronic records in UK primary care may threaten confidentiality, either in reality or in Anna's perception. On the other hand, the registration system and use of EHRs enables systematic monitoring and prevention of undesirable drug interactions. |

**Table 12.1** Continued

| Patient | Australia | Canada | UK |
|---|---|---|---|
| Daphne | During the pregnancy, Daphne has the freedom to find a GP to support her pregnancy, independent of her routine care.<br><br>The indemnity insurance situation in Australia means that she is unlikely to have a choice over the birth itself, which will be in a hospital Obs. & Gynae unit under the care of a consultant. | During the pregnancy, Daphne has the freedom to find a GP to support her pregnancy, independent of her routine care.<br><br>Daphne's options for the birth itself depend upon the province in which she is based. The birth is almost certain to be in a hospital and under the care of a consultant. However, midwifery care is included in public health benefits in some provinces, and available as private care in others. | During the pregnancy, Daphne has the freedom to use another GP in her registered practice to support her pregnancy, independent of her routine care.<br><br>She has a range of options for the birth itself, but whilst a home birth is available it is likely to be discouraged in a first birth, although more readily available in a second birth. A much larger role will be played by midwives and later health visitors. Doctors are only likely to play a significant role in the birth in the event of problems. |
| Harold | Unfortunately for Harold, orthopaedics is one area where waiting times in Australia are not much better than the UK. Even if he can afford the private premiums, he will not gain much in terms of waiting time.<br><br>On the other hand, he would be more likely to move to find a GP that suited his needs as this is much more common than in the UK. | Harold is likely to get his operation more quickly in Canada, although there is little systematic monitoring of waiting times.<br><br>As there is no private care, he will not be disadvantaged by his inability to pay for his operation. Also, he would be more likely to move to find a GP that suited his needs as this is much more common than in the UK. Doubt that changing GPs would make much of a difference for having hip op. | Unfortunately for Harold, elective surgery in orthopaedics is one area where waiting times in the UK are poor. As he cannot afford private insurance premiums, he would not be able to be treated privately to reduce his waiting time.<br><br>Although he has the option to change the GP with whom he is registered, there is considerable evidence that he is unlikely to do so. |

care and happily had health benefits as well. The UK health outcomes data during the 1990s provide evidence for this. However, there remain barriers to achieving further benefits in the UK and in other systems. In the UK, the inability to balance additional costs in primary care from prescribing (e.g. in asthma management) against savings in secondary care discourages care which is clinically and cost-effective. In Canada, the stumbling block is doctor remuneration. The PCR pilots in Ontario did not appear to be cost-effective as capitation levels were set at a level which would make province-wide roll-out prohibitive. In Australia, the emphasis upon patient choice and resistance to patient registration schemes seem to limit the role of primary care reform, although if the national prescribing record becomes a more general electronic health record then this may change.

- *Using primary care to improve health outcomes may destroy its value to patients.* Most of what currently happens in UK primary care and in Australian general practice is not advanced medicine. It is care of a more general nature which is highly valued by patients and has a big impact upon their quality of life. Primary care reform is seen by Government policy documents as the transfer of care from secondary to primary care. Secondly, primary care is seen as the place where data and information can be collected to assess health need and measure outcome. This has a range of potential side-effects for the more general and traditional primary care:
  - it will reduce time for patient contact by diverting time into data collection
  - it may damage the patient–clinician relationship by threatening patient confidentiality
  - these aspects may not be part of external targets used to influence doctors' performance
  - it may make the profession less attractive to doctors, increasing the current manpower shortages by encouraging early retirements and by discouraging recruitment.

- *The potential for dramatic and tragic failure remains.* The similarity between the problems experienced in the hospitals in Bristol, Winnipeg and Perth is disturbing. Further, the reaction of many UK clinicians to the events in Bristol and the subsequent reduction in public confidence has been a defensive one. This in turn reduces the likelihood of transparent behaviour in future, which is a necessary prerequisite for prevention of future disasters. The size and provincial/state structure of Canada and Australia has also reduced the opportunity for national lessons to be learned.

- *Healthcare policy decisions are driven as much by ideology as evidence.* Healthcare is undoubtedly highly political. As such, decisions, especially in the UK and Australia, have been driven by political ideology rather than good evidence. Interestingly, the UK Government is now starting to adopt policies which are not in line with its traditional ideology, e.g. foundation hospitals, PFI. Whether this reflects pragmatism or a fundamental shift in ideology remains to be seen. In Canada, whilst some political ideology emerges from the Provincial Governments, the split between Federal and Provincial Government means that no one ideology is dominant. Instead, the ideological position has been built up around the Canada Health Act. Even in Canada, where it is politically expedient, e.g. in the private provision of drugs, the Government has adopted a pragmatic position.

# A personal conclusion

Finally, the only way in which I can answer the question 'What is a good healthcare system?' with integrity is to express a personal view of what I have discovered in carrying out this work. In order to do this, I need to define my biases and values going into the project.

Coming from the UK in the aftermath of Bristol, Alder Hey and Shipman, it was inevitable that the problems within the UK NHS would be very apparent. The reforms of the NHS in the early 1990s had produced a degree of inequity in the UK system which also seemed a strong negative. This was exacerbated by the availability of private healthcare for those who could afford to pay for it.

By contrast, the Canadian system appeared to offer much better access to care and appeared much more equitable than the UK NHS. The fee-for-service system encouraged clinicians to provide a comprehensive service to patients and allowed them to spend more time with their patients.

On the other hand, the Australian system appeared chaotic and anarchic. The push to private healthcare insurance seemed to be driven by ideological rather than health reasons or even cost savings.

Having studied the systems, some of my views have changed. The UK system has a number of clear strengths:

- In spite of its problems, caused largely by a lack of resources and sometimes because of them, the system of patient registration and 'cradle-to-grave' care provides major benefits for patients and the management of their care, and a strong base for building a truly integrated and electronic patient record which can provide further benefits.
- The multi-professional approach to healthcare and the reduced primacy of the doctor offers significant benefits to patient care, especially in the areas of chronic disease, long-term care and ante and postnatal care.
- Following Bristol and other *cause célèbres*, the UK probably has the best monitoring systems, certainly of the countries examined. This, coupled with the culture change which allows clinical performance to be evaluated, is a major advance.

Against this:

- The latter systems, together with an increase in litigation, are in danger of promoting defensive clinical practice, which is not in the interest of the patients.
- Access to care, particularly elective surgery, remains extremely problematic, and capacity shortfalls will take a significant time to address. This is exacerbated by the availability of private care which perpetuates the inequity in the system and perhaps reduces the ability and incentive to raise the general standard.
- Management is becoming increasingly centralised and target driven. There is a danger that the greatest strength of the UK system – the cradle-to-grave* care – will be destroyed in the attempt to meet other targets.

---

*Some prefer the more graphic 'sperm to worm' description (quoted by Dr Nikki Shaw, amongst others!). In my view, these people have spent too long with their medical friends and colleagues!

The strengths of the Canadian system mostly stand up to scrutiny, although the absence of waiting time data makes comparison with other systems difficult. However, close scrutiny does reveal a number of flaws in the system:

- The exclusion of drugs and other services, such as home care and dentistry from Medicare, form an increasing source of inequity, which may start to be addressed following the Romanow report.[60]
- Primary care reform and moves towards more systematic clinical management of patients are restricted by the power of the doctors, their associations and the hospitals.
- Provincial variations and access to care in rural areas are also sources of inequity in the system.
- Provincial boundaries prevent national action on quality safety and regulation and therefore allow for the possibility of errors in one province being repeated in another.
- There is insufficient evidence to conclusively demonstrate that waiting times in Canada are satisfactory.

The Australian system remains something of a conundrum. On the face of it, it has all the disadvantages of the Canadian system together with the added cost and complexity of a public/private dual system. Whilst it is possible to provide much evidence that this does not provide an optimum solution, this must be balanced against the finding that most of the Australians that I talked to were far less angst ridden about their healthcare system than people in either the UK or Canada. This may simply be a national characteristic.

Alternatively, it may be an example of the thinking illustrated by Sir Humphrey Appleby in the classic BBC comedy *Yes Prime Minister*:[104]

| | |
|---|---|
| Sir Humphrey: | Bernard, what is the purpose of our defence policy? |
| Bernard Woolley: | To defend Britain. |
| Sir Humphrey: | No, Bernard. It is to make people *believe* Britain is defended. |
| Bernard Woolley: | The Russians? |
| Sir Humphrey: | Not the Russians, the British! The Russians know it is not. |

Similarly, the purpose of the Australian investment in private healthcare may be not to provide better access to care, but simply to make people *believe* that the healthcare is better and more accessible.

Against my initial prejudices, in spite of the evidence that private delivery *per se* does not improve healthcare performance or economy, and in spite of the evidence that the recent rush to private insurance has not improved matters, the Australian hospital system delivers very good access to care in comparison with the UK and probably Canada. Their primary care system remains a problem for this UK-centric author.

In a recent presentation, Dr Glyn Hayes[105] argued that the needs of the healthcare system appeared radically different if you were one of the 'worried well' rather than being seriously ill. This mirrors my distinction between basic needs and meeting patient expectations. My final conclusion would be that whilst I count myself in the 'worried well', the UK NHS seems to provide a solution. By the time I find myself in the category of the actually ill, I would rather be somewhere else, probably Canada.

# References and further information

To view the original material, visit the website that accompanies this book at http://www.goodhealthcare.org.uk where you will find links to most of the material cited.

1  These data were taken from the website of the International Caesarean Awareness Network. Whilst clearly a group with an agenda, the UK and Canada data were compared to the official government statistics and appear to be sound. These sources are available on-line and accessible through the Chapter 2 section of the website accompanying this book.
2  Hill K, Abou Zahr C and Wardlaw T (1996) Estimates of maternal mortality for 1995. *WHO Bulletin.* **79**(3): 182–98. This paper contains much on how the measurement was made as well as the actual data. It is available on-line and accessible via the website accompanying this book.
3  The UK Department of Health website waiting list data. Access via website.
4  McDonald P, Shortt S, Sanmartin C *et al.* (1998) *Waiting Lists and Waiting Times for Health Care in Canada: more management!! more money??* A report commissioned and published by Health Canada.
5  Statistics Canada data are available on-line and accessible through the website accompanying this book.
6  The Australian Institute for Health and Welfare data is available on-line and a link is provided through the website accompanying this book.
7  Access via website.
8  Orwell G (1948) *1984*. Secker & Warburg, London.
9  The 1978 Alma-Ata Declaration is available from the WHO website. Access via website.
10  Cambridge University rag mag, *c.* 1980.
11  National Audit Office (2002) *NHS Direct in England*. HMSO, London.
12  I heard Professor Robert Evans, University of British Colombia, expound the idea of a zombie at the 2002 Canadian Health Economics Research Association (CHERA) conference. It is referenced in the conference report.
13  Kaye JA, Melero-Montes M and Jick H (2001) Mumps, measles, and rubella vaccine and the incidence of autism recorded by general practitioners: a time trend analysis. *BMJ.* **322**: 460–3.
14  Wright C (2002) *Health Care Supply and Demand: maybe less is more*. Emmett Hall Memorial Lecture, CHERA 2002, Halifax, Nova Scotia. The complete lecture can be found through the website accompanying this book – there is a lot more in the speech.
15  Department of Health (1997) *The New NHS: modern, dependable*. HMSO, London. Available on the DoH's site, accessible through the website accompanying this book.

16  Health Canada (1999) *Canada Health Act Annual Report 1998–1999*. Health Canada, Ottawa, pp. 2–3.

17  Source of data: the Organisation for Economic Cooperation and Development. Available on-line and accessible through the website accompanying this book.

18  This paper is available via the website.

19  Source: Statistics Canada. Taken from Current Price GDP Income, 1961–1993.

20  The Report is available on-line and accessible through the website accompanying this book.

21  National Forum on Health (1998) *Final Report*. National Forum on Health, Ottawa.

22  Department of Health (1998) *A First-class Service*. DoH, London.

23  National Expert Advisory Group on Safety and Quality in Australian Healthcare (1999) *Final Report*. NEAG, Canberra.

24  Health Canada (2000) *Quest for Quality in Canadian Health Care*. Health Check, Ottawa.

25  Garvin D (1984) What does quality mean? *Sloan Management Review*. **4**: 125–31.

26  Crosby P (1986) *Quality is Free*, McGraw-Hill, Maidenhead.

27  Eddy DM (1984) Variations in physician practice: the role of uncertainty. *Health Affairs*. **3**: 74–89.

28  James B (1999) NSW Ministerial Advisory Committee: Quality in Health Care Workshop notes for training program for clinical leaders in quality management skills, 4–9 July 1999.

29  Ellis J, Mulligan I, Rowe J and Sackett DL (1995) In-patient general medicine is evidence based. *Lancet*. **346**: 407–10.

30  Fletcher M (2000) *The Quality of Australian Healthcare: current issues and future directions*. Occasional Papers, Health Financing Series, Volume 6. Commonwealth Department of Health and Aged Care. This paper is available on-line and accessible through the website accompanying this book.

31  Department of Health (1998) *A First-class Service*. HMSO, London. Access via the website.

32  Evidence given by Professor Chris Ham to the Commission on the Future of Healthcare in Canada (*see* reference 60). After this research was carried out and during the write up, the Romanow Commission on Healthcare carried out its work. Whilst it was not possible to include this in this stage of the work, the Romanow Commission report and research is referred to in the analysis stage. See reference 60 and read the final report of the Romanow Commission on-line, via the website accompanying this book.

33  A history of the NHS is provided on-line and a link is provided from the website accompanying this book.

34  Department of Health (1990) *The New GP Contract*. HMSO, London.

35  On the website you will find a discussion of the methodological implications.

36  National Audit Office (2001) *Inappropriate Adjustments to NHS Waiting Lists*. HMSO, London. Access via the website.

37  Protti D (2001) *Evaluation Report on Information for Health*. Department of Health Information Policy Unit, London. The entire report is available on-line via a link from the website accompanying this book.

38  Sowerby Centre for Health Informatics at Newcastle website, 2002. A link to this site is provided from the website accompanying this book.

39  Goddard J, Alty A and Gillies AC (2001) *A Case Study in Mental Health Informatics.* Proceedings HC2001, Harrogate, March 2001. British Journal of Healthcare Computing Ltd. The author of this study was a student of mine and can be contacted through me.

40  The Information Commissioner's guidance on healthcare is available on-line and is accessible via the website accompanying this book.

41  Hurley J, Vaithianathan R, Crossley TF and Cobb-Clark D (2002) *Parallel Private Health Insurance in Australia: a cautionary tale and lessons for Canada.* CHERA 2002, Halifax, Nova Scotia. This article is accessible through the CABOT database – a link is provided on the website accompanying this book.

42  The report is available on-line and accessible through the website accompanying this book.

43  Medicare Fact Sheet 6, *How Australia's Health Service Compares Internationally.* Doctors' Reform Society. The original can be viewed on-line via the website accompanying this book.

44  The Organisation for Economic Cooperation and Development (OECD) data can be accessed on-line via the website accompanying this book.

45  Anderson GF (1998) *Multi-national Comparisons of Health Care.* Centre for Hospital Finance and Management, Commonwealth Fund, Johns Hopkins University, USA. The newsletter uses data from this article.

46  The newsletter also uses data from the Australian Institute for Health and Welfare, available on-line via the website accompanying this book.

47  Evidence given by a representative from the AMA to the Commission on the Future of Healthcare in Canada (*see* reference 60).

48  Private Health Insurance Incentives Bill 1998, Second Reading Speech. The Hon. Dr Michael Wooldridge, Minister for Health and Aged Care. The text of the complete speech is available on-line and via a link from the website accompanying this book.

49  For non-Australians, Divisions of General Practice are organisations selling their support and advice services to GPs. To find out more, visit the website of a Division I visited in Melbourne, the North East Valley Division of General Practice, via the website accompanying this book.

50  Woodruff T (2000) The way backward in primary healthcare: corporatised medical centres [editorial]. *New Doctor.* **74**. The complete editorial is available on-line and accessible via the website accompanying this book.

51  Clarke R (1988) Just another piece of plastic for your wallet: the 'Australia Card' scheme. *Computers & Society.* **18**(1). This and an important addendum published in *Computers & Society.* **18**(3) are available on-line via the website accompanying this book.

52  BMMS Proposal, General Practice Computing Group, Royal Australian College of GPs, 2001. The full proposal is available on-line via the website.

53  BMMS Legislation, Department of Health and Aged Care, available on-line via the website.

54  Details of the Practice Incentive Programme can be found on-line via the website.

55  Details available via the website.

56  Historical analysis based upon data drawn from the interim report of the Romanow Commission on Health. A link to the report is available via the website.

57  The full Canada Health Act is available via the website.

58 Wright C (2002) Emmett Hall Memorial Lecture. CHERA 2002, Halifax, Nova Scotia. The full text of this speech is available on the CHERA website, accessible through the website accompanying this book.

59 Final report of the National Forum on Health, Volume II, 1998.

60 Commission on the Future of Healthcare in Canada (2002) *Building on Values: The future of healthcare in Canada – final report*. Commissioner: Roy J Romanow. The report is available from the Commission, accessible via the website.

61 Source: Alberta Government information on what is not covered by the Alberta Health Insurance Plan. See the information on-line via the website accompanying this book.

62 Visit the website of the Australian College of Midwives for more on this, accessible via the accompanying website.

63 Evans RG (1984) *Strained Mercy: the economics of Canadian healthcare*. Butterworths & Co., Toronto.

64 Deber R (2002) *Delivering Healthcare Services: public, not-for-profit or private?* Discussion Paper No.17. Romanow Commission on the Future of Healthcare. Available on-line through the website accompanying this book.

65 Health Canada and Ontario Ministry of Health Information, published on their websites and accessible via the main website.

66 Evidence given by Professor Cam Donaldson to the Commission on the Future of Healthcare in Canada (*see* reference 60). At the time Professor Donaldson was at the University of Calgary, Alberta. He has since moved to the University of Newcastle, UK.

67 This document can be accessed via the OMA website through a link provided on the website accompanying this book.

68 The Price–Waterhouse–Cooper evaluation report on primary care reform is available on-line and can be accessed via the website accompanying this book.

69 More information on the Ontario Family Health Networks is available from their website, accessible via the website accompanying this book.

70 Pong RW (2002) *Health Transition Fund Synthesis Series: rural health/telehealth*. The executive summary is available on-line and can be accessed via the website accompanying this book. Ideal for bureaucrats, pedants and insomniacs!

71 The full report of the Health Transition Fund 2001–02, accessed via the website.

72 Source: The Organisation for Economic Cooperation and Development, available on-line, accessible through the Chapter 9 section of the website accompanying this book.

73 ibid.

74 Department of Health (2001) *The NHS Plan*. HMSO, London. Accessible via the website accompanying this book.

75 To find out more about PFI, visit the PFI Network website, accessible through the website accompanying this book. The PFI Network has been developed by the Office of Government Commerce's Private Finance Unit to provide one-stop access to comprehensive information about PFI and assist the public sector PFI community to exchange information and to work more effectively.

76 Department of Health (2002) *Annual Report: 2001–02*. HMSO, London. Access via the website.

77 Wanless D (2002) *Securing Our Future Health: taking a long-term view*. Public Enquiry Unit, HM Treasury, London. Access via the website.

78   Department of Health Information Policy Unit (2002) *21st Century IT Support for the NHS*. HMSO, London. Access via the website.

79   Evidence given by Professor Ake Blomqvist to the Commission on the Future of Healthcare in Canada (*see* reference 60).

80   Evidence given by Professor Keith Banting, Director of the School of Policy Studies at Queen's University, Kingston, Ontario, to the Commission on the Future of Healthcare in Canada (*see* reference 60).

81   Commission on the Future of Healthcare in Canada (2002) *Building on Values: the future of healthcare in Canada – interim report*. Commissioner: Roy J Romanow. Provides great detail on CHST legislation. Access via the website.

82   Data from the Department of Finance is available on-line and is accessible via the website.

83   Kennedy I (2001) *Learning from Bristol: the report of the public inquiry into children's heart surgery at the Bristol Royal Infirmary, 1984–1995*. HMSO, London.

84   Taken from the Bristol inquiry final report (*see* reference 83). Read more about the terms of reference on-line.

85   Smith R (1998) All changed, changed utterly [editorial]. *BMJ.* **316**: 1917–18. Access via the website.

86   Redfern M (2001) *The Report of the Royal Liverpool Children's Inquiry*. HMSO, London. Access via the website.

87   The interim report (and the final report when published) of the Shipman Inquiry is available on-line via a link from the website accompanying this book.

88   The Commission for Health Improvement's website is accessible via the accompanying website.

89   Report of the Manitoba Pediatric Cardiac Surgery Inquest, 1998. The full report into the deaths of these children is available on-line via a link from the website accompanying this book.

90   Australian Council for Safety and Quality in Healthcare (2002) *Report into Obstetrics and Gynaecological Services at King Edward Memorial Hospital, 1990–2000*. Access via website.

91   Treasure T (1998) Lessons from the Bristol case. *BMJ.* **316**: 1685–6. Access via website.

92   Department of Health (2001) *Response to the Bristol Inquiry*. HMSO, London. Access via website.

93   The General Medical Council/Department of Health (2002) consultation paper is accessible via the website. Revalidation is described in detail on a website established jointly by the GMC and DoH.

94   Davies JM (2001) Painful inquiries: lessons from Winnipeg. *Can Med Assoc J.* **165**(11): 1503. Access via the website.

95   National Expert Advisory Group on Safety and Quality in Australian Healthcare, op. cit. Access via website.

96   Gillies AC (1997) *An Evaluation of the UK Fund-holding Experience*. 7th CHERA Conference, Ottawa, 1997. Access via website.

97   Department of Health (1998) *Information for Health*. HMSO, London. Access via website.

98   Department of Health (2002) *Annual Report: 2001–02*. HMSO, London. Access via website.

99   Evidence given by Professor Carolyn Hughes Tuohy to the Commission on the Future of Healthcare in Canada (*see* reference 60).

100 Evidence given by Claude Forget, former Health Minister, to the Commission on the Future of Healthcare in Canada (*see* reference 60).
101 Roy Romanow, in a speech to announce the final report of the Commission on the Future of Healthcare in Canada (*see* reference 60).
102 Department of Health and Ageing Press Release, November 2002. Access via website.
103 Source: Australian Institute of Health and Welfare. The data are available from the AIHW website, accessible via the website accompanying this book.
104 Lynn J and Jay A (1989) *The Complete Yes Prime Minister: the diaries of the Right Hon. James Hacker MP*. BBC Books, London.
105 Presentation by Glyn Hayes, Chair, British Computer Society, Health Informatics Committee, Burnley, November 2002.

# Index

Printed and bound by CPI Group (UK) Ltd, Croydon, CR0 4YY

23/10/2024

01777678-0005